TUMOURS

of the

BREAST

TUMOURS

of the

BREAST

And Their

TREATMENT AND CURE BY MEDICINES

By

J. Compton Burnett. M.D.

B. Jain Publishers (P) Ltd.
USA—EUROPE—INDIA

TUMOURS OF THE BREAST AND THEIR TREATMENT AND CURE BY MEDICINES

13th Impression: 2013

Published by Kuldeep Jain for

B. JAIN PUBLISHERS (P) LTD.
1921/10, Chuna Mandi, Paharganj, New Delhi 110 055 (INDIA)
Tel.: +91-11-4567 1000   Fax: +91-11-4567 1010
Email: info@bjain.com   Website: **www.bjain.com**

Printed in India by
JJ Imprints Pvt. Ltd.

ISBN: 978-81-319-0768-9

PREFACE

In common with a certain small number of other practitioners of scientific medicine in different parts of the world, I have long been in the habit of treating *tumours* of various parts of the body by medicines, and that with great success. When, a few days since, a young girl, whom I knew, was sent to a hospital for operation for a small mammary tumour that I am quite sure could have been cured by medicines, I felt it to be my imperative duty at once to bring my own views and experience more prominently to the fore, and the more so as our knife-men—our surgical carpenters—are waxing bolder and bolder every day, and the very excellences of aseptic and anaesthetic surgery are fast running legitimate medicine to the ground, and with it our common humanity.

I have been in spare moments occupied with a larger work on the amenability of tumours, wherever situate, to medicinal treatment, but I have not time to finish it at present, and as I had prepared what here follows of Tumours of the Breast as its first chapter, I am sending this to the printer as a smaller independent work. Of course this makes my present literary venture scrappy and rather disjointed, but I have thought the transcendental importance of the subject would overtop these defects of style and homogeniety. This much is explanatory merely. I have thought it well to give particularly my earlier and more difficult cases. They constitute a history of my gropings in the medicinal cures of tumours. I do this because they show the way in which I have come to light, and not because they are otherwise particularly instructive.

2 Finsbury Circus, London, E.C., July 9th. 1888.

J. COMPTON BURNETT

TUMOURS OF THE BREAST

By tumours I understand all lumps and swellings whatsoever the same being more or less growths on or in the breast, and *also* such as are usually called cancer. This work is not intended to deal with the causes of tumours beyond the merest outlines, as this subject I reserve to be dealt with by itself. I have great faith in "one thing at a time." Nor shall I dwell at every great length on my reasons for giving this or that remedy, because otherwise I should have to omit many of the details of the course of the cures related and because most of the indication are homoeopathic, and can be deduced from the proper pharmacological sources by any *competent practitioner who will take the trouble;* and these sources are medical literature in general—the literature of the homoeopaths more particularly, and specifically, the records of drug pathogenesy by Hahnemann and by his followers going back nearly to the beginning of this century. Some of the indications are, of course, empiric or hypothetic. Neither shall I make any attempt to give the pathology, of any given case further than shall be necessary to make it's name justifiable and it's nature comprehensible; but I distinctly state that cancer is included by me in the term tumour. It will thus be seen that the position I take is essentially clinical.

It may be asked, what do I give if I limit my indications to a few remedies, and say so little of the pathology of the tumours? I reply that my *object is principally to show,* TO PROVE BEYOND ANY POSSIBILITY OF DOUBT, THAT TUMOURS CAN BE CURED BY MEDICINES. And I do not travel all through literature to prove this propositions, but just content myself throughout the first clinical part with setting forth the out come of my own experience thereon in as few words as I can. Had I some new prompt and painless mode of excising tumours of the breast to bring forward, I should probably be hailed as a benefactor of the human race, yet without being anything of the kind; but as I advocate the divine art of *real* healing (and that mostly on heterodox lines), I must be content with my work as it's own reward, and, all things considered, not a bad reward either. Often when I have saved a breast, I have vividly before my mind the pregnant exclamation of the lady (*Diary of a Physician*) in regard to her ablated breast—"Ah doctor, but my husband!" A greater reward than to prevent this anguish of soul in some of my sister the world cannot offer me.

I declare that *the knife is no cure for tumours,* and that tumours can be cured by medicines, the requisite knowledge and *patience* being given. In order to be able to excise a tumour successfully, a man must first learn how to do it; it is the work of a skilled mechanic merely, in which there are many masters. In order to be able to cure a tumour by medicines, a man must also first learn how to do it, but it is the work of the patient chess player, in which there are but few masters. Still, without being a master, the art of curing tumours by medicines can thanks to Hahnemann and others—be learned and practiced by all in direct proportion to their ability and industry.

The great art in curing tumours by medicines may be thus summarized–*keep on pegging away*! Only, of course, we must peg away with the right remedies. Any medical person who reads this book attentively will have a good idea of how to set to work. I do not attempt or pretend to be in any sense apologetic or diffident or the question of the amenability of tumours to drug treatment, for the good and sufficient reason that I have been curing tumours by remedies for the past dozen years, and, therefore, I am discoursing only of what I know and have seen; that I have attained to my present certain position with much difficulty, endless gropings, and, I fear, some bunglings, goes without saying—*Ca va sans dire,* in fact.

The "Vicar of Wakefield," of glorious memory, says : "I was ever of opinion that the honest man who married and brought up a large family, did more service than he who continued single and only talked of population."

In like manner I am of opinion that the physician who sets about trying to cure tumours by means of medicines does more service to mankind and to medicine than he who only talks of how to cut them out, and of the microscopic and macroscopic characters and peculiarities of such growths after he has cut them out. Accordingly, I had not been in practice very long before I occupied myself with the question of the curability or noncurability by medicines of quite a number of diseases commonly called incurable, and amongst them *Tumours.*

The very first tumour I had to treat was a small hard one of the eyelid of some years' standing. The patient was a young lady from Canada. She had consulted an eminent physician of the homoeopathic school, and he had advised *an op-*

eration. "Have it cut out," said he, "medicines cannot cure it." She was sent to me by a mutual friend to see if I could cure it with medicines, and so avoid the dreaded operation. The tumour was but a small affair, about as big as a very small marble, but on a girl's lower eyelid that is a good deal. I used a number of remedies, but the two that seemed to be really curative were *Argentum-nitricum* 1, in one or two drop doses three times a day, and *Hydrastis canadensis* applied freely to the tumour with a camel's hair brush.

The little tumour completely disappeared, the patient and her people were enthusiastically grateful, and I made up my mind to look to my own experience in the future, and not think quite so much of the negative opinions of the supposedly great, for a very eminent medical father had said medicines could not cure this little lump, but I found medicines did cure it for all that. A good many years have passed since then, and I have been treating cases of tumour ever since with medicines, whenever I have had the opportunity; and when the patients have been as patient as their physician, have generally succeeded in curing them.

Of tumours of the eyelids I have succeeded in curing a great many generally purely constitutionally, but the very hard; *indolent* ones some-time need to be painted with the medicament, or to have it applied as an unguent, they being, as it were, outside the organism.

Some of the little tumours of the eyelids that one commonly meets with are from a wrong condition of the stomach, the state of the pancreas seems distinctly answerable for a certain number of them, some are apparently a sequel of vaccinia, and odd articles of food are known to cause them in certain people, e.g., roast pork. Often such swellings will rapidly disappear, but not in frequently they become hard, insensitive, and chronic. A few months of proper constitutional treatment will cure them. The remedies most commonly indicated are *Thuja-occid., Argentum-nitricum, Natrum-sulphuricum, Pulsatilla-nig., Hepar-sul., Calc., Hydrastis-canadensis.* In very obstinate cases one has at times to call in the aid of certain nosodes. One of the last cases of *tumours* of the eyelids I have had to treat, has only just got well after many months of persistent treatment with medicines, the patient being a young married lady whose husbands friends were very anxious for her to have them excised, but the lady would not listen to their entreaties, having been told by me that such tumours are of a constitutional nature, and must be treated constitutionally by internal medication. She was jeered at and ridiculed by the wiseacres of her husband's family for "being so silly." said they (*they knew* !) "Of course, you must undergo an operation. No medicines can touch *that.*"

For some months they seemed to be right, for my remedies did but very little good, and my poor patient had to bear a good deal of banter and "did not I tell you medicines were no use ?"

However, after a month of *Chionanthus-virginica* in small material doses, the tumours waned and went.

Said I, "What do your husband's friends say now?"

"Nothing !"

"Do they believe now that tumours of the eyelids can be cured by medicines?"

The lady passed out of my consulting room laughing.

In defending and fighting for unloved doctrines, I often see these positive refusals to believe SELF-OBSERVED facts, and I marvel at the cowardice of these *pretended* non-believers. I sometimes fancy that the reason lies in the fact of *their* not being the originators.

Less than two years ago, a child was brought to me suffering from paralysis and atrophy of a portion of the right lower extremity, that the local doctor said would end with the child's death in about a year or less. The most eminent London opinions, both special and general, confirmed this view. When the parents informed the local doctor that the child was to come under my care, he piously expressed the hope that it might avail, adding the rider: "If that homoeopath cures him, I will believe in homoeopathy."

When, however, the child was well and was running about on two straight, equal limbs, the said doctor looked very wise (what an easy task !) and stern, but would on no account have any conversation on the subject.

The amount of dense-mindedness and disin-genuousness that lies hidden in those WHO HAVE SEEN great homoeopathic cures and still resist the truth, must be immense. Though one rose from the dead they would not believe. Still, per-haps, I ought not to blame them, for it is very difficult to believe that medicines can cure tumours; indeed, there was a time when I could not have believed the contents of this book. I therefore desire to be charitable to others, being myself a Saulus and a Pulus.

THE USUAL VIEWS
AND PRACTICE

Two or three days after penning the fore going account of medicinal cures of tumours of the eyelids, I chanced to go to the office of a city solicitor or a matter of legal business. "Ah, doctor," said he, "I have been away for a fortnight from business. I have had an operation on my left eye; just look. I have been at home a fortnight with it since. I had to keep it bound up".

On looking at his eye I saw nothing abnormal, and I said, "Your eyes are all right." I then found that he did not differentiate between eye and eyelid, and that he had been operated on for a tiny cystic tumour of the eyelid!

Said. he, "Mr B, did it for me, I am all right now."

The gentleman he referred to is considered, and indeed is one of the first ophthalmologists (eyecarpenters) of the day, and the solicitor, I may say, stands well in his own profession; so we may take them both as fair samples of the educated professional classes of to-day. In other words, a layman with a trained mind gets a little lump on his eyelid, FROM INTERNAL CAUSE, as I submit.

He merely wish it removed with the knife, as if it had dropped from the sky, and had impinged upon his "eye." He goes to an eminent oculist – what more neutral? And said oculistic chirurgeon being on the same general educational and physiological level, gains in every way by cutting out the little cyst!

Both the individuals concerned have not the faintest suspicion that they are other than the *crème de la crème* of all that is most advanced in knowledge, and in the every van of progress. They will die in the happy delusion, and their work and names will not be remembered.

Did I try to enlighten my slicitorial friend by explaining that in as much as the said cyst was autochthonous, it ought to have had it's existence cut short autochthonously?

Did I explain to him that the cyst was a qualitative outcome of his organismic, self and that this self-same microcosmic should have been put right vitally?

Did I ? No.

Why ? Because you cannot put a large quantity into a small vessel, whether the vessel be called surgeon, solicitor, or beer glass.

Of the tumours of the eyelids, the meibomian cyst is very common, and also very amenable to medicinal means. It will once in a way disappear of itself without and medicines, but not very often; usually it must be got rid of either by operation or medicines. The usual way is to reverse the lid, and make a small incision from the inner lid surface which cover the tumour, and then squeeze out the contents. But "the tumour is likely to recur." Says a very experienced operator! Of course it is !

In my opinion, the encysted and other tumours of the eyelids are nearly always of constitutional origin, and must be constitutionally cured.

I will not burden my book with any more preliminary cases of tumours of the eyelids for introductory purposes. The bulk of them are not only curable by remedies, but the task is not even a very difficult one, though at times a little tedious.

Tumours are very common in the breast, particularly, in women's comparatively rare with men in this region.

I will now go on to my special task by citing a more formidable case—one of genuine cancer, cured by *Condurango,* a remedy which I proved on my own person a number of years ago, an account of which may be found in *Allen's Encyclopaedia of Pure Materia Medica,* Art. C.

I will merely call it a HARD TUMOUR OF LEFT BREAST.

In the spring of the year 1875 I was treating the children of a family of my *clientele*. While chatting with the children I noticed that their nurse, a women of about forty, had an ugly unsightly *crack in the left angle of her mouth,* about the fourth of an inch deep, and surrounded with warty excresences, the whole covered with a nasty secretion I considered it commencing epithelioma. I offered to treat the woman for it, but she did not believe in homoeopathy, and she was using a salve to it prescribed by her own doctor. At this period I was myself still suffering from my proving of *Condurango (see British Journal of homoeopathy,* July 1875), and I had repeatedly proved that the crack in the angles of the mouth was a very characteristic symptom of the drug. Altogether I have seen it produced pathogenetically four times, and I have cured along many times. It apparently find no favour with the profession, but it's importance will be recognised.

Some little time elapsed, and the before mentioned nurse was confronted with the chance of losing her situation, as her mistress was getting afraid lest the disease might be communicated to the children. The nurse was now willing to be treated homoeopathically, and her mistress accordingly sent for me. On inquiring I found the warty ulcer in the angle of the mouth was only a little worse; it was very *torpid,* had remained for many months, pretty much the same. This is also characteristic of *Condurango.* The pustules and other cutaneous manifestations of this drug are torpid (see the proving in the *British Journal of Homoeopathy and the* "Symptomatology" in *Allen's Enyclopaedia of PURE Materia Medica,* vol. iv., p. 1 et seq.) Once while using an ointment this ulcer had almost disappeared, but it soon returned to the condition I have described.

But what alarmed both mistress and maid (the former on account of the children, no doubt) was a *tumour in the patient's left breast i.e.,* on the same side as the epitheliomatous ulcer of the angle of the mouth. On examination it was found to be about the *size of a small hen's egg, and very hard* and very painful at times; at other times painless. It had been there for several years, and was on the increase, but only very slowly. The odour from the axillae was very offensive indeed, but not from lack of cleanliness. Speaking generally, patient did not look ill-nourished or cachectic, though her teeth were very badly decayed, which gave an old appearance to the face from the falling in of the cheeks, and the dilated small cutaneous blood-vessels showed that she had probably been a florid subject.

The *history of the tumour* was this. She had four years been in the habit of sleeping with the youngest child, a bonnie boy, with a very large, heavy head, and he lay with his head against this breast. To that she attributed the lump. And she was probably right, for the boy would at times restless at night, and hit about with his head a good deal, hence we may fairly conclude that the breast had been mechanically injured very many times. Patient complained that he very often hurt her thus.

There was nothing to account for ulcer of the angle of the mouth; it was idiopathic, as the phrase goes. There could be no reasonable doubt of the connection existing between the tumour and the ulcer. Was it cancer? I think so now, and I thought so than. I do not *call* it a case of cancer, but simply a tumour of the breast, hence my diagnosis cannot be called in question, whereas if I were to *call* it cancer it might be objected to. Still I will say I think it was cancer,—1st, From the appearance of the floor and edges of the ulcer; 2nd From the coincidence of the ulcer and of the tumour; 3rd

From the hardness of the tumour; 4th From it's origin.

It is needful to state this view of it's pathological nature, as it influenced the treatment.

The medicine I decided on was *Condurango,* and for these reasons:

1. *Condurango,* produces cracks in the angles of the mouth, and also cures such.

2. *Condurango* is in my opinion, an antipsoric, and case appeared to be a psoric manifestation from injury.

3. *Condurango* has beyond any doubt cured cases of cancer, and this seemed such a case.

4. It seemed to me that the ulcer in the angle of the mouth that started more crack-just supplied the pathogenetic differentia requisite for knowing whether to give Hydrastis, Conium, or what not.

The first prescription is dated July, 16, 1875, and is

Rx Pil. *Condurango 1*, 3ij

One four times a day.

This was taken until December 4, 1875, when

I could perceive only slight amelioration of the ulcer and none of the tumour. I then remembered that the cures reported had been with material doses, and that Goullon, jun., and another writer on the subject on the Continent, whose name has escaped me seemed to incline to that view. Now, I would rather cure a patient with a big dose than leave him or her *uncured* with a small one. And, of course, conversely.

Moreover, my patient rather objected to pilules; the size of the *means* seemed so *inadequate* to the *end*. Therefore I gave the following preseription, in December 1875:

Rx Tc *Condurango* θ 3ij

Aq. Ad. Zvj.

C.c med. ter in die.

This was taken till September 1, 1876 with slight interruptions. At this date I certainly noticed much improvement in the ulcer, and the tumour seemed a little smaller, but still I felt very much disappointed. Then *Bryonia-alba* 1, two drops in water four times a day, was given till November 10, 1876 when, no further progress being apparent, I gave a short course of *Sulph*. 30 one pilule at bedtime. This is very old practice, and has been verified a great many times. In all about one drachm of the pilules was taken. Then at the end of 1876 I again went over the case and felt justified in reverting to the old prescription of *Condurango* but I gave the tincture of the first centesima dilution three times a day with occasional omissions, that the organism might not get insusceptible of the action of so small a dose. This was continued during the whole of the year 1877 during the first months of the year 1878, and during the first five months of the year 1879 that is just about two years and a half. I saw the patient at, intervals during this period, and was able to observe the course of the cure. In a few words it was this. At first the ulcer of the angle of the mouth became dryer, cleaned and less rugged, while the tumour went smaller and a little. About a year and a half the ulcer had entirely cleaned and remains so; nothing happened but a very slight puckering, of that angle of the mouth and faint streaks of scar-tissue. But to a casual observer these objective symptoms have no existance, it is only when examining it critically in the light of it's past history that one can detect even these trifiling rests.

Already towards the end of the year 1878 the tumour had nearly disappeared, and in the spring of 1879 it was gone. In sending a Report from Princes Park, Liberpool on September 2, 1879 the patient says :- "The lump has completely gone out of my breast," Further she goes on to state that she gave up taking the medicine. This case is very important from various stand-points; it shows the utility of proving a remedy that has an empirical reputation in order to find out the variety of a disease that it will cure. Thus *Condurango* has undoubtedly cured a number of cases of cancer; but we may say the same of *Sulphur,Thuja, Arsenicum, Conium, Hydrastis, Carbo-animalis, Bryonia, Bufo, of Galium Aparine,* and hence the point to find out is what characterize or species. The greatest characteristic yet observed of our *Condurango* is the crack in the angle of the mouth, and hence on theoretical grounds we may say that a case of cancer with a manifestation in the angles of the mouth calls for *Condurango*. Now we have one such case on record as cured.If my readers will not admit that it was cancer well, I have no objection.

This case is strikingly important from another view, viz.. it illustrates the torpidity of the *Condurango* variety, and it also teaches most valuable lesson to us all. Never despair! This woman patiently took her medicines for four full years, and now she has her reward in health, and I have mine in the comforting consciousness that I did not listen to a very able physician who pooh-

poohed the proving of *Condurango,* and who ridicules the idea of curing tumours with medicines. As J. Stuart Mill says, "He who knows only his own side of the case, knows little of that" I may add that when I last saw the patient she had very much improved in general appearance, being stouter and fresher, younger.

NINE YEARS LATER

published the foregoing case in the Homoeopathic World, November 1, 1879, and I have just made inquiries regarding this woman, who was thus cured of her tumour, notwithstanding its declared impossibility, and find that she still continues in perfect health and free of tumour.

A certain number of distinguished practitioners of scientific medicine (homoeopathy) have from time to time published cases of tumour as cured by medicines, but these cases are on record, and need no further writing about. I therefore will not refer to them, as my object is not to bring together odd cases of tumour cured here and there all over the world, some of them quasi-accidentally, but to bring new clinical material to the general stock. I have not time to collect these strewn-about cases in our literature, however in-

teresting and instructive the task might then,
perhaps, get at some fixed indications, though of
these clinical fixations I have heretofore met with
but very few. In these pages, therefore, I purpose
giving my own experience solely-just some facts,
and these I leave to tell their own tale.

One thing I may say-it is quite useless to try
to cure old tumours either cancerous or benign,
unless you are gifted with PATIENCE of no ordinary kind. Rapid cures of old tumours by medicines I have never seen, nor do I think such tumours
ever will be cured rapidly, simply because they
are vital products-THEY ARE LIVING GROWTHS.
Nevertheless it will be seen from the cases which
I shall presently narrate, that some recently-
formed tumours do get well in a very few weeks
or months. While other require as many years.
Speaking broadly, the tumour takes proportion-
ately as long to cure by medicines as it has taken
to grow. And hereby is not to be forgotten that a
tumour has often existed a long time before it is
found out. It is equally useless to try to cure
tumours by giving drugs with a view of dissolving
them chemically.

Why ?

Because, as just stated, tumours are ALIVE
: they are GROWTHS; they come via vita, and
vitally they must be cured ; and for this process

time, often much time, is needfull. At least that is my experience, and I therefore specially emphasize the fact, that I know of no short cut to tumour-curlng., by remedies, and the work must be done by internal remedies.

Nevertheless, externally applied remedies are not to be entirely neglected, i.e., where the growth is for any reason, as it where, extra-organismic. Where I use a remedy externally I shall state, the fact, which, as will be seen, is rarely the case.

Derivatives I also occasionally use, and also, temporarily, tonics. But let me proceed with my facts.

In case I should subsequently omit to state the fact, I would say that pig-meat, milk, much salt and pepper, are, In my judgment, to be avoided in tumours of the breast. New milk is particularly bad for mammary tumours and inflammations, as also for menstrual troubles.

TRAUMATIC SWELLING OF RIGHT BREAST CURED BY BELLIS ALONE

adduce the following case of a swelling in a young lady's breast, particularly to exemplify in a neat way the curative range of the

DAISY in the treatment of tumours.

No experienced practitioner, will deny the important part played by bruises, blows, and falls, in the genesis of tumours and cancer ; and hence our anti-traumatics ought to figure much more largely in our therapeutics of growths from blows. Before giving my case I will quote a very instructive note on this very question that appeared as leader in the first volume of hole Homoeopathic Recorder (Philadelphia), No. 4, July 1986.

It turn thus :

MALIGNANT GROWTHS

In the preceding number of The Recorder there appeared three items concerning malignant growths, which deserve more that passing notice. One is the history of the development of a malignant formation as the result of the frequent mechanical irritation of a simple mole on the face, another recounted the cure of an extensive sarcomatous growth by an intercurrent attack of erysipelas, and the third contained the analysis of a series of cases of carcinoma, in all of which there was antecedent injury by mechanical or chemical means; in the later selection the writer asks in all seriousness : Is cancer, whatever its form, ever primary, i.e., does it ever originate without previous injury ?

A negative reply to this inquiry is of the highest importance to those who believe in the curative effects of drugs. It deprives the disease-action of part of the mysterious, fateful quality so constantly associated in our minds with these affections, and which terroixes to some degree the powers of the medical attendant. For, we hold that the great majority of physicians, on discovering the existence of a suspicious growth, are strongly impelled to advise the use of the knife as the only sure treatment, not with standing that in case of undoubted malignancy, the value of surgical interference is greatly lessened by the relatively poor results as measured by the added years given to the patient.

Moreover, if the occurrence of an infectious inflammation of the skin has destroyed malignant disease-process in that tissue, there is a fairly good basis for the view, reasoning by analogy, that a drug-disease, i.e., a disease produced by the action of a medicine, can, if affecting a part involved in the malignant process, cause similarly efficacious results.

In an admirable Report* on the Progress of Pathology, by J. H. Muser, M. D. Mr. Sutton, F.

R C. S. is given as authority for the following view ; "Irritation, local or otherwise, affecting the tissue, may cause abnormal epithelial growths which, rising above the general level, may produce a wart. On the other hand, the epithelial growths may dip into the sub-.epithelial tissues, and on account of lack of formative development either from decline of vigor or general constitutional debility, the new tissue never develops functionally, runs riot, and originates tissues of low vitality-car-cinomata. The conditions favourable to the development of carcinomata-debility, etc.-are absent in the young we have warts; in the old cancers."

What, then, is the bearing of these facts upon the treatment of probably malignant tumours ? Passing by the cures of warts by internal medicine alone, which almost every homoeopathic practitioner has observed over and over again, we need only call attention to the cures, by the same method, of tumours of the female breast, an organ notoriously disposed to malignant neoplasms; here the action of Conium cannot be densed and what true of this remedy may be true of many others.

A thorough study of the symptoms of each individual case the view of finding the exact simillimum, the exhibition of the letter in different attenuations, if necessary, changing the remedy only when a change of symptoms demands it, and extreme watch fulness for involvement of the neighbouring glandular structures, make up it appears to us, the duty of the physician. Whether he would be justified in holding out any hope of cure by internal medication after evidences by systemic infection exist, must be decided by his own experience, but, as there are always cases in which it will not be allowed, opportunities will not be wanting to continue treatment with the properly chosen remedy.

If statistics of our treatment can be collected and analyzed, the results will, we feel sure, give encouragement to physicians and suffers as well, and demonstrated anew, and in strikingly brilliant manner, the value of our law of cure.

We earnestly hope, then those of us who hold hospital or dispensary appointments, will endeavour to employ the method of internal medication in cases of malignant growths, whenever it is fairly admissible to do so, and that records of cases containing diagnosis checked off as to their accuracy by every method known to medical science, together with the symptoms in full and the treatment used, may soon appear in our journals. Thus will be laid the foundation for a new and lasting monument to homoeopathy.

Without going so far as the author of this article, I must certainly say I attribute some of my success in the treatment of cancers and other tumours by medicines to a due recognition of the traumatic fact, not in diagnostics merely, but also in therapeutics.

Miss L.C., aged thirteen years, came under my observation at the end of July 1879. About eight weeks previously a miserable lad in the street hit her in the right breast with considerable violence ; from that time this breast became swollen and very painful, until at length she was quite unable to lie on her right side. Patients mother was poitrinaire, as was also her brother, and my experience teaches me that the members of poitrinaire families are particularly liable to suffer from blows.

At first no notice, was taken of the young lady's complaints, but week after week went by, and she persisted in referring to the pain in her breast. I do not now remember, but eventually I was sent for, as vague notions of tumour and cancer rendered the parents useasy. On comparing the breasts, the right one was found to be by much the larger, being swollen and very tender.

I thought this is very proper case for testing the anti-traumatic virtue of the old English bruise wart, and hence prescribed thus :

    Rx Tc. Bellidis perennis 3x, two drams.

    S. Three drops to be taken in water four times a day.

    The result was a very rapid disappearance of pain and swelling, and in a fortnight patient could lie again on the right side. And a few days later an examination showed that the swelling had entirely disappeared.

    Nothing whatever was applied to the part, no change was made in diet, mode of life or place of abode and as the thing had already existed for eight weeks, the positively curative effect of the Bellis can hardly be denied which is the one point this case is meant to exemplify and to teach, and that because it is very difficult to demonstrate positively the effect of any one remedy when the tumefaction has become a genuine or hyperplasia.

    I published, not long ago, a book entitled *Fifty Reasons for being a Homoeopath,* and the foregoing was my forty-fourth reason.

    As I am here illustrating the curative range of Bellis perenis in the treatment of lumps of traumatic origin, I cannot retain from dragging in a very late experience of mine with it, though it has really no right at all to be here, being not a tumour of the breast at all but a TUMOUR OF THE JAW.

A gentleman at the prime of the life, or a little beyond some might think, came to me at the end of 1887 with a hard tumour in the right upper jaw of about two years standing. It had come on slowly. His dentist thought it was due to a set-up tooth in the wall of the jaw. An eminent surgeon had seen patient with the dentist, and was not of the dentist's opinion, believing it to be a new formation, for which he prescribed an ointment containing Iodie (la vieille histoire !) The ointment dutifully applied, and did no good.

The right half of face between eye, mouth and beard was notable swelled hard, and with glistening, shiny skin over it. Regarded front within the cavity of the mouth, it appeared as if the outer wall of the antrum Highmore were pushed out, constituting a tumid mass.

All things considered, I thought the dentist right and the surgeon wrong, and, on the mechanico-traumatic hypothesis, gave Bellis per. Q, five drops in water night and morning, and two months of this brought the jaw back pretty well to the normal, and patient did not think it needed any further special treatment. Nor indeed did it, though to my eye the right upper jaw looked a tritle fuller than the left, but a few months later when I saw him I could not see any difference in the two sides.

These two cases having been cured in a very short space of time, apparently contravenes my previous statement that tumours cannot in my experience ever be cured quickly, I therefore add that this evidently was not a neoplasm, but merely mechanical obstruction with slight incipient circumuscular hypertrophy of tissue. Tumours of a neoplastic nature come by growth, and can only be cured by atrophy, and vitally and not chemically, and so the progress must in that case be shown. Of course we should theoretically expect a tumour that was of long duration to take more time of a congestive nature with only incipient hypertrophy; and with this the oretical expectation my practical experience entirely coincides.

TUMOUR OF RIGHT BREAST; TUMOURS OF RIGHT ARM; ARM-PIT; SEVERE CUTANEOUS AFFECTION.

The case I propose now to narrate has taught me much in respect of the amenability of mammary tumours to drug treatment.

Indeed more than any other one case in my whole experience, and I may, perhaps, be therefore permitted to dwell upon it a little fully, more particularly in regard to it's causation. The subject of it came under my medical observation in the year 1878, and she was then verging on 40 years of age. An examination disclosed several lumps in the right axilla about the size of a goose's egg, and all hard.

It appeared that the tumours in the arm-pit had been there for two years, and came after a successful vaccination; and simultaneously therewith, the face had broken out all over with an eruption of ruberous inflammatory elevations, with pustular stop technically termed acne variolae formis, and this eruption has also persisted for two years in this very aggravated form, like chronic small-pox. In the year 1877 there was an epidemic of variola in the neighbourhood, and patient was again vaccinated, so her vocation brought her into contact with it, and this time it was followed by the lump in the right breast. I did not then regard vaccination as a causal factor in the genesis of chronic disease, but I see now clearly enough that it was a case of chronic vaccinosis, axillary and mammary swelling and the facial eruptions being clearly of common nature and origin. An operation was not thought useful by her rather open minded friends, and hence my help was sought I treated the case for a long time with such remedies as *Silicea, Psorinum, Sulphur, Hekla-lava, Grauvogl's Lapis alb., Conium iodirum, Phytolacca dec.,* but made no great headway. The lady was, however, very patient, and went on with my treatment, feeding principally on hope; but hope, though not a bad auxillary, is no remedy for tumours or skin disease. I then used various so-called nosodes, sometimes utilized by homoeopathic practitioners with isopathic procivities, and we made a little progress, but not much. When however, I had obtained more correct views of the long-lasting effects of the vaccinial poisoning, I prescribed *Thuja-occid, Sabina, Vaccinium* and *Variolinum* in varying dilutions (mostly medium and high), and patient slowly got quite well, not only of the adenomata in the axilla, but also of the tumour of the breast and of the skin affection.

When she was up in London for the May meeting in 1888, the lady called upon me, and thus I am able to say that she remains perfectly cured.

Never have I seen a case that so well exemplifies and justifies my principle in regard to the treatment of tumours—Keep on passing away!

That this lady would have died long since had she been operated on for the tumours I have no doubt at all. Others may doubt this, but that she was cured of her tumours by medicines is open to no doubt whatever. Amongst the frequent causes of tumours I must, therefore, reckon vaccinosis, and on this subject I would refer the reader to my little treasise entitled Vaccinosis and it's Cure by Thuja* etc. in which this thesis is to some extent elaborated. Sometimes we have to do with trauma upon vaccinosic tissue, and then the just appreciation of the two genetic factors leads to a cure.

TUMOURS OF LEFT BREAST
AND OF RIGHT OVARY

On Februray 5, a married lady, 40 years of age, came to me borne down by the weight of her physical miseries. Her father had lupus of the nose, and her mother had died of cancer. Eight years previously a very small tumour had been excised from patient's left breast and now there is another in the same breast. In addition to their tender swelling. The right ovary and the left breast are, curiously alternate in painfulness, tenderness and several trouble sameness. Patient's first baby was born dead, after very protracted labour. She had also suffered from sore throat, leucorrhoea, piles, thick scanty urine, and then profuse and limpid; stricture of the sigmoid of the flexure at it's lower end, much pain in the breast and side, rectum packed full of piles, sore throat, worse in the night, and by far the most distressing symptom of all, constipation of the most severe and obstinate kind. Patient made two conditions to my being her physician—the first was that I should allow aperients; "Life is unbearable without them." Said she; and the second was that I should tell her what each given remedy was, "because I take so much interest in these things." I absolutely declined both conditions, and the patient yielded, but under a desperate running fire of sarcastic obstructiveness, consisting in diffusive and effusive epistles, such as your clever lay *guerisseues homoeopathiques* so well know how to keep against a stiff-necked medical autocrat, little weaning that mental obedience is an essential part of the cure of some cases. However, she did give way slowly, and was eventually rewarded by being completely cured. At her visit to me on October 20, 1886, she well of tumour, of stricture, of piles, of constipation, of all pains (and of all the other physical miseries formerly complained of. The treatment lasted over three years, and the remedies used were in the order named):

Aesculus hippocastanumt 3* trit.

Sulphur 30.

Nux-vomica 30.

Graphites 4 trituration.

Psorinum 30.

Thuja-occidentalis 30.

Lapis-alba (Grauvogl's) 4 trit.

Mercurius (strength not noted).

Silicea 6.

Graphites 5.

Silicea 6.

Besides various well-known and less well-known nosodes, the cure was aided a good deal by diet.

And in regard to diet, I think I could hardly do better than quote a very opposite paper by a very gifted lady, the late Mrs. Nichols; it will be found further on. I will produce it, as it is almost unique in it's scientific purity, and in dietetics the scientific spirit is almost entirely absent; most doctors, I notice, go by their own stomach or old wives tales, as witness the rubbish one hears and reads about vegetable diet.

CANCER OF BREAST

In the year 1883, a London professional man was under my care, and in odd conversations he told me about his mother who had cancer of the stomach. Could I do her any good? I did not know, probably not.

I saw him pretty frequently. And almost every time after I had prescribed for himself, he recurred to the said state of his mother and her terrible sufferings, dreadful pains in the chest and stomach, keeping her awake at night for many hours together." She had her left breast removed some time ago for cancer, and now it had come in the right breast and in the stomach.

Could nothing be done ?

I told him that I often succeeded in curing simple tumours with medicines, and also cancerous tumours of small size if taken early, but that when they had one been operated on I mostly failed, the operation apparently generalized the disease and intensified it, so I could not give him much hope. Had she come before any operation had been performed, it would have been very hopeful.

So time went on, and still my patient insisted

on conversation with me about his mother, of whom he is very fond. He even stopped me at railway stations to tell me of the poor lady's sufferings. Finally, en desespoir de cause, he brought her to me for my opinion. I am now particularly pleased that he did so, as the course of the case taught me for the first time the vastly important lesson, that even after an operation we need not give up hope,— nay, more, that where an operation has been performed, constitutional treatment should be begun at once, to get at the root of the matter and prevent any further local expression of the disease, by attaching it's cause or cause. I say or causes, for cancer is not a disease that can produce it's like after the manner of, say syphilis or scarlatina, but is essentially a hyperlasia of a degraded type at the end of a chain that has many (causal) links. But to may case :

October 23, 1883. Mrs.—, 47 years of age, had her left breast removed for cancer two years ago last. May by an eminent surgeon. In February 1883 she had erysipelas of the face, and as she lay in bed therewith paresis of right foot, which passed off. She had variola at the age of three; is subject to winter bronchitis with much dyspnoea. On examining the chest, one sees a long but very neat scar where the left breast used to be. The other and inner ends of scar are a little tender, and the tissue at the outer end is rather swollen of late. The patient cannot bear the part to be touched. The right breast is the seat of a hard painful tumour of the size of a hen's egg. The pain, however, is worst in the stomach (the ventriculus), which pain is "cruel," like cramps, and worse at night.

Rx Tc. *Condurango* 1x,, four drams. Five drops in water three times a day.

November 16. Only had two attacks of stomach-pain since she was here. Anorexia no better; much flatulence; "flying spasms."

Rx Repeat.

December 12. Much better in herself; stomach pain gone; had it a year; pain in the toe no better; the mammary tumour in less hard.

Rx Repeat.

February 6, 1884. Menses at first stopped, and patient gave up the medicine, as she attributed their cessation to the medicine; after leaving it off for a fortnight she got menorrhagia gets nocturnal dyspnoea; wakes up with a cough; stomach continues better; feet are sore; the appetite is now good.

March 28. Has been laid up with a cold and

bronchitis, but the nocturnal dyspnoea is much better; digestion fair; feet less sore; the pain in the stomach has not returned; the tumour is very much softer.

Rx Tc. *Silicea* 30, four drams. Five drops in water night and morning.

April 28. The tumour of right breast is decidedly less painful; there is now a hard painful portion of tissue over the site of the left breast, which pains most at midnight; patient feels ill.

Rx Psorinum 30

May 5. Feet very tender; both breast and the painful tissue very much better.

Rx Tc. *Hydrastis-canadensis* 1, four drams. Five drops in water three times a day.

June 11. Menorrhagia every fourteen days; feet very tender; tumour softer.

June 26. Has prolapsus recti, with constipation; dirty brown leucorrhoea; breast is painless; tumour smaller; no pain in the stomach; feet better, less painful.

Rx Tc. Thuja 30.

July 23. Worse; very much pain in the stomach; last night it was most severe; tumour hard and painful.

Rx Tc. *Condurango*1x, four drams. Ten drops in water twice a day.

August 20. The tumour is rather smaller, but more painful; severe pain in the stomach. Patient had gone back to the lemons which I formerly recommended, and which seemed to suit. There are now two painful nodes on the edges of the scar of left breast. Has had menorrhagia twice.

Rx Psor 30 and *Condurango* θ.

September 5. About the same; feet very tender.

Rx Tc. *Condurango*θ and Silicea 6 trit.

October 15. Feet no better; stomach well; no pain in the scar; tumour in the breast is smaller and softer.

November 10. Tumour of the breast much softer; the vaginal discharge has now ceased. Pains are always at night.

December 26. Much better altogether.

Rx Repeat.

January 7, 1885. Gone back very much; breast very painful; the submaxillary glands are swollen and painful; the pain is "cruel," and causes "vomiting by the hour;" vomits blood; pain keeps her awake at night; she has a taste of phosphorus in the mouth. She tells me now, for the first time, that she is an enormous pepper eater, which I forbid.

Rx Repeat.

Feb. 21, 1885 Been to the seaside to pull up; the natural pain is much better; the feet are tender and swell.

Rx Repeat et Cond. θ.

March 4.   Much better; right breast much more elastic; the   nipple is still very much retracted.

Rx Psor.c. et Cond.

April 30. The pains wake her up; she shrinks from pressure on the chest.

Rx Ranunculus sceleratus 3x. Four drops in water night and morning.

May 4. Has much pain under left arm, where there is some swelling nd redness.

Rx Bellis p. 1.

Rx Lapis alb. 5 trit.

June 17. Tumour decidedly smaller and better both sides.

July 22. Parts very tender, and there is much acidity.

Rx. Acid hippuric 6, four drams. Five drops in water night and morning.

August 28. Did her seemingly much good for three weeks, when she had a dreadful attack of a pain.

Rx Repeat (12).

October 21. Did her much good.

Rx Tc. q. Kreatin 12, three drams. Three drops in water night and morning.

November 20. Much better; in fact, nearly well, but has whites now badly.

February 5, 1886. Has not been since November 20, 1885. She says the powders than given gave her cramp in the stomach, waking her up between 12 and 2 A.M., and causing nauseous risings; pains in the feet, which are sore and tender. Left them off, and the same phenomena recurred on resuming them. Has had no medicine for a month, and these symptoms persist. When she has a stool, the faecal mass slips backwards in the rectum.

Rx Trit. 6, *Silicea* gr. vj., ter die.

March 17. The breast is nearly normal, but the womb and feet are painful.

Rx Repeat.

May 5. Womb and feet better; gums very spongy, much water-brash and vomiting of water.

Rx Tc. *Natrum muriaticum* 12, four drams. Five drops in water three times a day.

June 28. Says the drops have very much upset her; gums are very blue.

September 4.

Rx Aconite and *Silicea.*

November 2. Breast well, gums still red and swelled and sore. Much abdominal pain from 2— 4 A.M.

Rx Trit. 4, *Urea* gr. vj., ter die.

Patient has paid me irregular visits off and not since, for gouty pains in various parts, but there no return of the cancer.

I have given so many tedious details this obstinate and difficult case to illustrate several points as clearly as I am able. In the first place, this case caused me to modify my previously oft-expressed opinion, that when once an operation had taken place, treatment by medicine is useless. I now know that this is not necessarily the case, but that a cure may be obtained even after an operation, and after a recurrence has begun. In the next place I again learn, and continue to insist upon, the importance of dogged perseverance in the medicinal treatment. And finally, it confirms my general practice of striking out new therapeutic lines when the old ones do not suffice. The influence of the late Dr. Ameke's, teachings will be readily recognised by the learned in pharmacological and therapeutic offshoots.

Looking now back on the whole of this case, considering all it's points, the remedies those helped and those that did not I get a comparatively clear view of it's nature, which helps me in other case. Were I asked to name it's biopathology, I should say it was a hybrid union of psora, vaccinosis, chronic poisoning by pepper and tissue-gout, to which complexity there came the element trauma.

MAMMARY TUMOUR

n July 5, 1883, a lady of 73 years came under my observation for small hard tumour in her left breast. This breast had been injured thirty year ago, and gave her much trouble

for long time. For some months she has noticed
it's swelling and hardening. It pains a good deal;
worse at night, and on moving the arm. In the
preceding November there had been an eruption
on the patient's left leg, "large inflammed patches
showed themselves." The principal remedies used
were Bellis-perennis 1, Psor. 30, Var. 30, Hydrastis 1, and then finally Bellis I again; and on January
29, 1885, patient was discharged cured; and she
remained well, and is, I believe, alive and well at
the time of going to press.

I do not give the details of this case as it is
badly kept in my diary, but the foregoing contains
most of the essential points, and the fine pharmacologist will readily see that the prescriptions were
all more or less ex hypothesi. I might add that
patient is deeply pitted with small –pox marks.

HARD PAINFUL TUMOUR OF BREAST

On August 13, 1878, Mrs.—, a country
clergyman's wife, between 40 years of
age, came under my care for a tumour of the left
breast in it's outer and upper aspect. It about the
size of the very small hen's egg, hard and very
painful. It had existed for some time, and she and
her husband had become very anxious about it,

the more so as her mother had died of vulvar
cancer (an enormous epithelioma). Perhaps I ought
to say that the mother died with the cancer, as
she was 82 year of age at her death. The mother
had been my patient, but she was, she averted,
unable to persevere with my medicines (Thuja 2,
3 and 30) as they caused her so much pain.

Patient is married, has several fine children,
and has been long subject to a very severe form
of leucorrhoea.

It would occupy too much space were I to give
all my notes of this interesting case in detail, for
she was under my treatment for this tumour about
three years.

My notes begin with August 13, 1879, and
prognosis was a serious one unless medicines could
be made to prevent the disease advancing.

I began with Urkalk gneiss 4th trituration,
ten grains at bedtime, and soon got into trouble
on it's account, for my patient showed the prescription to a learned lay lady, who is the recognised
stock-taker general of all the unfortunate leeches
of the neighborhood in which they dwell, and she
said, "Oh, Mrs.—know what the doctor thinks you
have the matter with you it's cancer!"

"How do you know?"

"Oh, the chemist told me it was the new German cancer medicine."

Naturally this caused my patient much and needles anxiety, but then the chemist and the learned lady must have their confidenatial little whisperings about the doctor's doings—it is no inconsiderable part of their rather monotonous lives. But this and many other similar experiences have compelled me often to withhold the name of the remedies.

Well, Mrs—took Grauvogl's Lapis alb. (4, 5 and 6 trit.) For a number of months without any noticeable effect; the lump went on growing, and the pain getting worse.

July 26, 1879. Acid. Acet. 1.

August 28. No better; very weak. Conium-maculatum 3x .

The remedy was continued for about two months, and it look away the pain, but it did not lessen the size of the tumour. Then followed Carbo. An. 30, which was suggested by the profound adynamia.

November 28. No pain; and she is no stronger, but the tumour is no smaller.

Rx. Sulphur 30.

On January 6, 1880, I received a letter telling me that the powders were finished, and that in addition to some pain in the tumour, patient had a good deal of pain in the stomach. I sent *Condurango* I. and ordered her to take six drops in water three times a day.

Feb. 24. "A good deal of pain and uneasiness in the whole breast and shoulder and down the arm."

Rx Repeat.

April 10. No. change in the tumour; "for two or three weeks I did not feel it at all, and now I have a good deal of uneasiness, though no acute pain."

Hydrastis I. Five drops in water night and morning.

May 19, 1880. On this day the lady was brought by her husband to London, and they called to inform me that having continued my treatment ever since August 1878 their friends wished for another opinion. The lady herself did not wish for any further opinion, but the husband was rather needlessly loud in demanding the opinion of at least one other, and that of Sir James Paget.

To this I declined to assent, because, said I, "What is use of an opinion, or for the matter of that, what is the use of a barrowful of opinions? The tumour is there; you can feel it and see it; that it is hard you can also feel; that it pains your wife knows but too well, and what possible prognosis can the men of the knife give but the everlasting old story, "Oh, you must be operate upon as soon as possible." Truth to tell, I am sick and weary of the lying statements that the knife is even any, and least of all the only cure for tumours. Not only does the knife not cure, but any one having a tumour or lump cannot, as a rule, take a shorter road to the grave than via the knife—that, is unless it be very large, and unless the tendency to it's recurrence be outrooted simultaneously with the operation, or soon thereafter.

Oftener than not, cutting out a small tumour is like pruning a vine.

But to return to my patient and her choleric husband, I absolutely declined my second opinion.

Why ?

Simply because a very considerable number of people with tumours literally die the doctors' opinions, and then what is the use or value of the opinion of a never so eminent a pathologist on a therapeutic point? Just none.

Of course, I know it is said to be very unprofessional to decline an eminent colleague's co-operation in a given case. But I did it for my patient's good, not for my own; and moreover, they do the same to me when people want my opinion.

Under date of May 19, 1880, I find in my case-book, "She has suffered for many years from white sticky leucorrhoea very much like the white of an egg; the tumour is softer, and about one-half it's original size; the whites are considerably better since the last medicine (Hydrastis 1x, gtt. v., night and morning). The tumour is more painful eight days before menstrual period.

July 20. Whites worse; more pain in the tumour; pain in the epigastrium, making her feel quite sick, especially when standing.

Rx Thuja 3, four drams., gtt. v., bis die.

September 16, 1880. It brought out an eruption.

Thuja 6.

November 16, 1880 Have been almost entirely free from pain until last week, when the breast pained me; I am much better in regard to the white. So far as I can judge, the last medicine has been the right one."

Thuja 12, four drams., gtt. v., bis die.

January 28, 1881. "I have taken the last medicine for two months. When I first began to take it, I had more pain in the effected part than I had had for a long time previously, but lately I have been quite well, except a spell of toothache, which yielded to Belladonna and Gelsemium. The tumour is very much smaller.

Rx Hydrastis can. I, four drams., gtt v., night and morning.

March 25. "I am going on improving, indeed I am very seldom reminded of my ailment; the tumour is now so small that my husband cannot find it."

Rx Hydrastis can. 6, gtt. v., four drams. Night and morning.

May 27. "After I began to take the last medicine I felt a good deal more uneasiness in the affected part than I had done for some time before. Now I am much as I was while taking the previous medicine. I think my husband told you of the decrease in size."

Rx Psor. 30, four in twenty-four hours."

July 29. "My husband thinks the lump nearly gone I think it is gone. While I was taking the last medicine, and for a week after, I had a good deal of pain in the region of the womb, and at the time

I had this pain I was also a good deal annoyed with the whites; now I am quite free."

July 29, 1881, is the last note of the case in my book but I saw the patient on another matter on November 3, 1886—more than five years thereafter—and learned that there had been no return of the tumour or of other ill-health, and she had enjoyed very good general health.

TUMOUR OF LEFT BREAST

rs.—26 years of age, came under my care in February 19, 1883, complaining of the swelling in her left breast about the size of a small orange. It was hard, and had been first noticed in August 1882. Last spring she had squeezed out some fluid from the left breast. Slight leucorrhoea. She was the mother of one child which was then three years old. Patient had been twice vaccinated, and was subject to labial herpes.

I informed the lady that the tumour was, in my opinion, due to her use of modern preventive measures, that it was, in fact, due to reflex irritations from the hypogastric region. My wide experience teaches me that a large number of mammary tumours in comparatively young married ladies are due to hanky panky manoeuvers of various kinds, the organism being, additionally, dyscratic. Without any dyscrasia, the hypogastric irritation would in all probability not so easily suffice, unless indeed, it were very great and applied over a long period. I explained that nature in the long run is very rarely insulted with impunity. Nemesis may tarry, but she inevitably follows the trail of wrong doing Oh, how true it is that the way of the transgressor is hard.*

Rx Psor.30.

March3. The tumor is rather smaller. She says, "I find it decreased by about one-half."

Rx Repeat

March 19.the tumour is a trifle larger than it was last time. The old itching has entirely disappeared.

Rx Kali chlor. 6 trituration, in six grain doses night and morning.

April 2. *Emansio mensium :* she is probably *enceinte.* Herself she feels rather weak, but the tumour has much diminished.

Rx Tc. *Thuja occidentalis* 30.

---

* "Man draf das nicht vor keuschen ohren nennen."
"Was keuschen Horizen nicht entbehran koennen."

Patient needed no further treatment, the tumour quite disappeared, and in due time a baby came.

UTERINE FIBROID; SMALL TUMOUR ON LEFT BREAST—DISEASE OF LEFT NIPPLE

n unmarried lady, 43 years of age, came under my observation on September 24, 1881, for a severe sprain of the left ankle. It was several months before she got well, it being complicated by gout, dyspepsia, and dysmenorrhea. The accident was severe fall down stairs, and, in falling, she struck with great violence against the low part of the body, causing for many months much vesical trouble with metritis. The case was further complicated with attacks of breastpang, and with fainting fits. Evidently the fall had given her a rude shaking, and disturbed many important organs, the liver and spleen giving at times much trouble. This lady remained under my care, and very slowly got the better of most of the just described ailments, when, on March 14, 1882, she took me so far into her confidence as to tell me she had, for the past four years a little red lump on her left breast that discharged something. It was about the size of a hazel-nut, and situated at the lowest outermost part of the left breast. With it there was much pain all down the left side.

At her next visit on April 19, 1882, patient took me further into her confidence, and started that she had been for some time getting very large in the uterine region,—in fact, the size had been noticed by strange ladies, who thought she was married, and was expectant. On this account alone the position was most painful. The case went on, the abdomen continued to increase in size, when, on November 23, 1882, I came to the conclusion from an examination obtained with much diffi-culty, that it was a uterine fibroid. The mammae became greatly hypertrophied. I could never quite make up my mind where are fibroid really sat, and sometimes from the hard nodes of the cervix uteri, I opinioned it might be a kind of fibrous hypertrophy of the whole organ. Very many rem-edies were used—Lappa major Q Thuja 30, Merc. met. 30, Lapis alb. 3, Aurum met. 100, Helonin, Kali chlor. 6, Aur. Mur. 3x, Silicea 4, Bovista 3x, Psor. 30, but all with but little apparent effect. Moreover, the left nipple became the seat or most distressingly painful moist cracks, and which are particularly significant.

This brings the case down to August 1883, when patient appeared like a lady about seven or eight months gone in the family way. To make matters worse, a child ran against her (impinging on the protuberant abdomen), and hurt her a good deal, when I gave Platin mur. 3x, but also to no good purpose. Any wonder that patient was getting down-hearted ? Two years medication and bigger than ever! And the doctor—Are a few guineas any adequate reward for such responsibility? Than came Bovista 3x, Mer. Cor. 5, Aur. Mur. 3, Helonin 3x trit., when the breast was a good deal better, the cracks of the nipples better, and the little tumour drying up. The excoriation between the legs was described by the patient as dreadful; pain in the back very bad; disagreeable taste.

Rx Lapidis alb., 6 trituration.

January 10, 1884. About the same in a general way; complains dreadfully of her back. This dreadful back distress finds grand remedy in the virus of variola, which I gave in the 30th dilution, and in very infrequent doses; and any one objecting there to answered thus: Aux grands maux les grands remedies.

February 14th. Seems to have done her back real good; left breast is much better; was so well that she absented herself for a few days. The same remedy was continued.

March 6th. Maintains that last prescription did her harm, while the previous one did her much good, which I can well understand, viz., de trop of the right remedy, back exceedingly bad; much frontal headache.

Rx Trit. 6 *Calc. Fluoris.*

April 5th. Head better; back very painful when she walks. Anorexia; bad nights.

26th. Has had a good deal of pain at the menses and in the left side, nights much better.

Rx Var. C.

May 29. The nights continue good; much easier in general; is getting thin; was very stout, notably mammary hypertrophy; is very debile, but the tumour is decidedly smaller.

Rx Tc. *Aur. Mur. nat.* 3x. Two drops in water night and morning.

July 10. "Dreadfull sicky," i.e., intense nausea; she feels very weak; tumour is much smaller.

Rx Psorinum 30.

August 21. Frequently faints away, at times falling down; less nausea; vision is failing.

Rx Thuja occidentalis 30.

September 6. Is still giddy, but does not actually faint away; has menstruated three times in eight weeks: sick feeling gone; dreadful pain in the left side; toothache.

Rx Argent. Nitric. 5, four drams. Five drops in water night and morning.

October 16. Much enlargement of the spleen, which pains a good deal.

Rx Tc. Ceanothus Americanus 1x.

November 5. No better.

Berberis vulgaris θ.

January 9, 1885. Breast well; the tumour of womb still very large; and patient has every appearance of being enceinte; wakes very early, and cannot get off again. (This is a capital indication for Bellis.)

Rx Tc. Bellidis perennis I.

Jan. 29. She now sleeps well, and feels much easier in the abdomen. I would here interpolate a rather important clinical tip in regard to Bellis, viz., it is often curative of the symptom, "Wakes early in the morning and cannot get off again;" and in cases of pregnancy and of uterine tumours (also enlarged heart), Bellis given great case, i.e., take away the effects of mechanical pressure.

February 26.

Rx Variol 30.

March 26. Back is on the whole better; tumour rather smaller; giddiness.

Ib. (C.C.)

May 9. Pain in left side.

Rx Ceanothus Americanus I.

June 8. Toothache and pains in the back.

July 23. Much pain in the left side. Which is tender. Tumour is smaller, which is evident from general appearance.

Rx Tc. Chionanthus virginica θ.

September 3. Side better; the left nipple is very sore.

October 2. The nipple is better, more comfortable; the tumour of womb about the same.

Rx Trit. 4, Hekla lava.

December 5. Feels much free from pain, and more easy and comfortable in herself than for long. This remedy has cured her constipation.

Rx Repeat.

January 26, 1886. Is very giddy; fairly comfortable in uterine sphere; left nipple has been gathering. She is so cold in her stomach.

Rx Tc. Kedron I.

March 9. Feels dreadfully sick.

Rx Trit. 3x, Hekla lav.

May 29. Patient is so much better that she is getting very irregular in attendance. The diminution in the size of the tumour is considerable.

Rx Repeat.

August 6. Continued marked improvement in the size of tumour, but there is a good deal of pain in her legs, worse on getting up out of bed in the morning.

Rx Tc. Bellidis per. I, Four drams, five drops in water night and morning.

October 6. This is the date of my last note when patient presented herself normally menstruating, in blooming health, plump and ruddy, though still complaining of some tenderness of the left ovary and left nipple. One can see where the little tumour formerly was on the left breast by the deeper colour of the skin. I prescribed Kali chlor. 6, which, no doubt, has taken away the tenderness complained of.

This is the long weary course of my treatment

of this terribly complicated case, lasting, as the notes show, just five years. During this long period my patient was very often importuned by her well-meaning friends and relations to undergo an operation, but she steadfastly refused, wavering only once or twice when her homoeopathic friends also urged surgical interference. If patient should call again before this goes to press, I shall add a few words more. Patient subsequently came to know if she might accept an offer of marriage, which I answered in the affirmative.

May 15, 1888. Patient continues well. I give it as my opinion, that had this lady been treated surgically, she would have died long since, and that miserably.

It is not merely medicines that will cure tumours, but diet and suckling will also do so. Let me give the following case, and to which I have previously referred.

TUMOUR OF LIVER CURED

BY MEAGRE DIET

In the *Herald of Health* Mrs. Nichols, a very talented lady, has been giving a retrospect of her own life-experience. The following portion has a moral, medical and scientific value:-

"I think that much of the sympathy I feel for the sick is due to my own ailments. If I had been born a strong child, if I had not known so many of 'the ills that flesh is heir to,' I should never have been a physician. I have loved my profession only because it has enabled me to relieve suffering—to reach the sickness of the soul, often through that of the body. Long ago I became convinced that all sickness is from sin—from voluntary or in voluntary disobedience to the laws of life. It is not the sin of the individual alone, but the sins of progenitors that afflict us with our many diseases. The study of disease and it's causes is the study of the human race, it's passions, it's sins, crimes, sorrows, and agonies.

"I have had my aspirations. I have loved literature and art. I have loved for a life of beauty, of abstraction from the sorrows of this earth life, but sickness of body and soul was born with me—with my humanity; for when I had suffered and had learned a way of relief, how could I refuse to help others?

"I did not study the art of healing in any ordinary way. I learned the science of cure in my own person. To illustrate this statement; I was

borne with disease of liver. No matter what part
of a parent is weak or diseased, of that weakness
or disease the child will partake. The child is
specially made from the mother. It the paternal
element is strong, it takes hold strongly upon the
maternal, but what the mother has not, that she
cannot give. If she has weak lungs or liver, fragile
bones, her child has the same in greater or less
degree.

"I inherited from my mother a diseased liver.
When a young child I remember (for my memory
reaches to my second year) bilious disorders which
caused me intense suffering. Of course I knew
nothing then, except that I was ill; and my parents
knew no more than I did. For ordinary illness they
used domestic remedies—tea made of tanzy, oak
of Jerusalem, mother-wort, etc. for serious illness
the family doctor was called, and his practice was
servere and sanguinary. Bleeding, calomel, jalap,
opium, antimony, etc., formed the Materia Medica
of my childhood. An empiric named Thompson
protested against bleeding, and introduced emet-
ics of lobelia and stimulus of capsicum, but the
first robbed the blood of it's serum to reject the
poisonous lobelia, and the last was little better
than drunkeness, the capsicum being prepared
with spirits, and a servere irritant in itself.

"The tender mercies of all medication were cruel in those days. If any pessimist says the world does not grow better, I have only to say to him. Look at the diseases and medication of fifty years since. As much blood was shed by lancet as in a war, and mercury was found impacted in it's crude state in the bones of patients who had taken the orthodox doses of calomel. The world is very bad in this 81st years of the 19th century, and much of it's medication is a cruel and unwise thing, but Homoeopathy is a fact, and water cure is widespread as prophylactic or remedial and the power of sympathy is recognised by many.

"The diseases liver which formed a part of my evil inheritance became so bad in 1868 that I sought the resistance of a learned water-cure physician. Certain reasons prevented a diagnosis, and I was thrown back upon myself to try what I could do for my relief of cure, as the event might be. A tumour had formed in the liver, so large that it had to be supported in the daytime by an elastic band, and in the night by a pillow. I had not rest, and scarcely any sleep. At about 5 o'clock in the morning I slept a little while. I could not take food without great distress. Digestion was never begun under seven hours, and only accomplished after hours of torment. In this condition I resolved to take but one small meal in the 24 hours, and that mid-day. I began this practice, and the third day I was so weak and giddy that my husband begged me to take some food. I was convinced that I must die if I took food, and I could only die if I did not I therefore resolved to rest what I could in bed, or on a sofa, continue my fast. I took one meal at mid-day; and when thirsty drank lemonade or orangeade. This I took in the forenoon, and I found it refreshing and not hurtful, a week from the beginning of my fast I slept well six or seven hours in the night. My spirits rose to cheerfulness. I was weak, and my working time was a good deal a bridged. I could work after my dinner, but I little in the forenoon but endure my weakness and a passionate longing for food. This however, gave way after a time, and my greatest suffering was from weakness and inability to work. For six months I kept this fast; only taking a moderate meal at mid-day, and sometimes a glass of lemonade or orangeade in the forenoon.

"At the end of six months, one day I took breakfast and dinner. The consequence was a burning digestion that made me more miserable than I can describe. Only once was I seduced into eating a breakfast. I continued my fast for another month, and the tumour on my liver was gone. It had been so large as to be felt by any one from the out side, I was now entirely dissipated, so far as I could judge from internal feeling and external examination.

"I now began to take a very light breakfast of bread and fruit, and little milk and water, and I made my dinner about seven hours after. This I have continued to do with good results, for the years that have elapsed since my cure. My digestion is slow, and I find that two meals a day suit me better than three. I have sometime varied from this course when away from home, but have uniformly found my health and digestion better when I have returned to the two meals a day, taken seven hours apart.

"I have had a great deal of practice in disease of the liver, and what are called 'Indian livers.' Much oily food causes and exacerbates hepatic disease. I have found in such cases a diet of whole wheat meal bread, porridge, and a half pint of milk for breakfast, and another half pint at dinner with fruit, only a little whole wheat-meal bread or fruit for the third meal most beneficial.

"We give hot-air bath where the patient can bear it, and the half pack and night. Sympathetic remedies and *Hydrastis canadensis* we have found beneficial. The kneading, or movement cure, and judicious exercise, are most useful. But of all remedies the diet is most important. Oily food of

all kinds is disastrous for diseased liver; neither
chocolate nor cocoa are admissible. To keep the
bowels free and open with brown bread and fruit,
and to use packing, or hot-air bath, to throw off
the retained waste and diseased matter, are very
important. In some diseased conditions of the liver
there is great constipation. The retained waste
matter is diffused through the system in the effort
to eliminate it, and it forms often the basis of
typhus. The use of hot air, or sweating pack, to
cleanse system is therefore all important.

"It will be seen from my narrative that the
tumour, or what some call lumps in the liver, can
be dissipated entirely. From of my seven months'
fast, I have never had an hour's suffering from by
liver.

Although this work is intended to give my
own experience only in the medicinal cure tumours
of the breast, I think the foregoing personal narrative of the sufferer herself eminently instructive. Some of the statements I do not quite agree
with, and I think the power of diet is often much
over-rated, still the subject to omit such an excel-
lent personal testimony. My objection to diet by
itself lies in the fact that many are too weak to
bear dieting, and very rigorous diet uses up normal tissue as well as morbid. I know of no case

of tumour of the female breast cured by diet, but I lately had the following case under observation, and in exemplifies the wisdom of Nature's own little ways, that some of the soft pated and sinful moderns are trying the upset. Only concelated soft-patedness would dream of throwing Nature's efforts.

ON THE CURE OF A SMALL
ADENOID TUMOUR OF THE BREAST
BY SUCKLING

lady of 32 had a little adenoid tumour in her left breast of the size of a marble. As she was enceinte, I recommended her to do but little for so small a thing, but to be sure to well suckle her child when it came. This she did with very praiseworthy prserverance, although she did with very little milk, and the process had to be materially supplemented by the bottle, and at the end of the 4th mouth of suckling the tumour had entirely disappeared. It is true I gave her few medicines also with reference to the tumour and for her ailings, still I conclude that the baby helped to draw off the tumour, casually of it waning; the mammilla of that side had always been retracted, which a small circumstance, deserves attention.

Personally, were I a woman with baby, I would suckle it from purely selfish motives, merely to departure my own blood and organism, for woman who has a family and does not suckle her offspring, is drawing a bill on the future of her organism which she is likely to be either unable to meet at all or to do so with great difficulty. Mother Nature suffers no tempering with her provisions; with her it simply and emphatically, obey; or suffer disease or extinction.

TUMOUR OF BREAST

The case I am about to tell is psychologically and sociologically interesting, as may readers will see.

On December 15, 1884, a married lady, 44 years of age, mother of one child, then 16 years old, came to place herself under my care.

She had noticed a swelling in her right breast, a was naturally much frightened. An intimate friend of hers (in fact, her former governess) had been cured of a mammary tumour by me with medicine, and so Mrs.—came off to London to place herself under my care, but when arrived, her metropolitan friends quite laughed her out of it, telling her it was all nonsense to trust herself to my tender mercies,—first, because of my homoeopathic proclivities, which they adequately despise and actively hate; and then "it was well known that no medicines (and least of all, homoeopathic once) were any good at all in tumours." The poor frightened thing of course yielded, was hurried off to what I suppose I must call eminent men, who declared it to be cancer, and urged immediate operation in order to save her life. The operation was duly performed in April, the whole right breast being completely ablated by Sir———. The wound healed up quickly and well, the lady was sent home to her husband's country seat CURED (!!) and the case, no doubt, continues to stand as one of the CURED(!) of the eminent operator. The social value of these quasicures by the knife is—baronetcy. The social value of medicinal cures of tumours is—slander and contempt.

However, the cutting-off process was worse than useless, as in a few months another tumour appeared in the remaining breast, which confirmed the opinion of the operator that it was a case of cancer.

Was it cancer ? No. I think not, but an irritable tumour of uterovarian origin. Indeed, I am quite sure this is the correct diagnosis. Our operating surgeons are mad; the biggest and best are clean mad. No sooner does a poor woman get a lump in her breast than she is frightened out her wits by consulations between these eminent and eminently ignorate knife-people, whose diagnostics are confined to feeling, seeing, and the microscope.

My treatment of this recurrent tumour lasted three years, and the following remedies were used—*Psor. 30 Hydrastis Canadensis q, Bellis per. I, Ranunculus sceleratus 3x, Psor.C,, Thuja occidentalis 30, Bellis perennis q. Solanum tub. 6 and 12, Aurum muriaticum nat. 3, CondurangoI;* and on February 7, 1888, the breast was normal, and the remarkable thoracic hyperaesthesia had at last disappeared, and this had for years been so bad, that the gentlest touch of one's finger on patient's chest caused her to wince and shrink from contact.

To all the notes of these three years of treatment would fill a little volume, and so I am compelled to narrate in the few words. But I again state that it was not a case of cancer, but the lumps came in the breasts—first in the one that was cut off, and then in the remaining one—from a wrong state of the uterus and ovaries, and in precisely the same physiological way as the milk comes into the breast after child-birth.

The origin of the first tumour was curious; the lady was getting out of their carriage when she fell against one of the buttons of her husband's coat. When I first saw the left breast it was red, hard and very painful. The lady had been vaccinated four or five times, the last twice unsuccessfully. She was very fond of salt. She had had much grief and worry. Her confinement was very severe, owing to size foetus. She subsequently had a good deal of congestion of the womb and leucorrhoea, for which her surgeon and physician gave her local treatment. This is the usual thing: at first a poor lady's constitution is wrong; Nature, kind clever Nature, sets about righting it with leucorrhoea, ulcerous at the os uteri, and uterine congestion; the doctor (poor brainless creature) cauterzes, gives injections, and cures (drives back); then in concretes in the breast as a tumour, which is cut off, and—apresca le deluge!

I told the lady straight away that hers was not a case of cancer at all, but as she had the opinions of the greatest living authorities on tumours and cancers she did not believe me.

What do her husband, family, and friends

now say of the diagnosis and the cure by remedies? I do not know, I merely have been made aware that they now poke fun at the duration of the cure. "When are you going to leave off going to your doctor ? Surely you are well, you look it ?" And these were the very people who prevented her from coming to me in the first instance, and morally compelled the poor frightened lamb to have one of breasts ablated !

When I was a student and used to watch my professors paint tumour with iodine, give their bearers tonics, fail to do any real good, and then explain authoritatively how that medicines were useless in tumours, and how that nothing but the surgeon's knife was of any real avail; when I used to see and listen to all this, I often dreamed day dreams of trying to find a solvent for tumours, and to avoid the cutting business, of which I have, and ever have had, and instinctive horror. And in the beginning of my professional career I tried hard and long to find such a solvent for tumous, but of course, never found any.

Why ?

Just because the thing in impossible. And why impossible ? Simply because the organism GROWS tumours vitally, and anything that is to cure, really cure must bring back the perverted

VITALITY of the part of the normal, and, fortunately, the semeiology and symptomatology of the sufferers, when read in the light of homoeopathy, give us good stout hand-rope to guide us in our search for the right remedies.

If we reflect upon the subject, we shall readily come to the conclusion that the attempt to cure tumour by locally-applied absorbents or by operation is like trying to cure an apple-tree of it's apples by painting the apples with iodine, or performing an operation on the apple-tree for "apples." The only difference the two process of apple-growing by apple-trees, and tumour-growing by human organisms, lies merely in the fact that the apple growing is a part of the normal biology of the apple plant whereas the growth of tumours by the human body is morbid.

This difference is, of course, a very great one, but what I am driving at is to show that tumour-growing is, though certainly morbid, yet nevertheless quite as much a vital process as if it were purely a biological process within the four corners of the normal physiological life of the individual. Gardners tell me also that the real seat of the growth of apples is roots of the tree, and that in the smaller lateral roots. Of that I have no personal knowledge, but I affirm, as the outcome of my own though, observation, and experience, that growth most tumours in the female breasts has it's rootings in the ovaries and womb. Of that I has no manner of doubt. This naturally does not apply to traumatic tumours of the breasts arising from direct blows on the breasts, but to a vast majority of all the others which are idiopathic or autochthonous.

MULTIPLE TUMOURS OF BREAST

An unmarried lady of 32 came under by observation on the 24th February, 1885 for a number of hard tumours in both her breasts, which were otherwise of enormous size, yet shapely. She had also prolapsus uteri, leucorrhoea, an enormous liver, the left lobe of which reached down almost to the navel.

Carduus Mariae q restored the liver to the normal, and so made more room for the dislocated womb, which soon took advantage of the altered topography of the abdominal contents; in fact the prolapsus was gone. Quite a number of nosodes followed in high dilutions, and then *CondurangoI, Chionanthus virgin θ, Helonias dioca θ, Hydrastis canadensis θ, Bellis perennis, Acidum fluoris 6, Fluoride of Ammonium 5, Secale cornutum 6,*

*Sarza θ. Solanum tub. 6, Scrofularia nod*osa 6; and, under date January 17, 1888, I find noted in my case-book-The breasts are quite normal, with the peculiar resilient elastic feel of that organ when healthy.

I attribute the original cause (or at least one of the causes) to numerous cauterization of the os uteri to which the unfortunate lady had been subjected by a fashionable lady's doctor of the repute. I do not mean that the cauterzations of the womb alone produced the tumours of the breast, but rather that what was the cause of the ulcers, being denied an outlet at the os uteri, became vitally concreted in tumid masses in the breast, aided by the reflected mammary irritation from the os uteri.

I feel it is not fair to my subject to give a string of remedies that were used to cure this case, without the same time giving their diagnoses and indications, but space fails me. I might just add that the most striking, prompt and permanent amelioration wrought in this case was by the Solanum tuberosum and by the Scrofularia nodosa, both in daily doses of five drops of the tincture of the sixth centesimal dilution, though the last prescription was the former remedy in the twelfth centesimal

CANCER OF RIGHT BREAST

At the beginning of the year 1887, a lady friend and patient was consulting me on account of her health, and she was very depressed and frequently burst into tears, I pressed her to tell me the cause of her grief. "Oh," said she, "I have a sister who is coming home from Germany to be operated on for cancer of the right breast. We all very fond of dogs, and one of my sister's dogs jumped upto her and hurt her right breast very much, and now it has turned to cancer. She has been using ice compresses for over a year, and been under the Crown Prince's physician, and under Dr. ——, who is sending her home for the opinion of Dr.——."

"It is there nothing in the world that can cure cancer ?" said she.

My reply was—what I here solemnly restate—that most cases of cancer are quite curable by the remedies IF TAKEN EARLY, AND TREATED LONG AND CONTINUOUSLY BY INTERNAL REMEDIES, and that in this way I had myself cured many cases of cancer.

"Then," said she, "I suppose it is too late for my sister, for she has had it for more than a year and a half, and the doctors say that the operation is her only chance."

April 2. I went to see the lady at her sister's house soon after her arrival from the Continent, and found them all very naturally, in a sad state of mind. The patient had received a letter from Dr— urging an immediate operation, as otherwise the cancer-juice in the milk ducts would infallibly poison her blood. Subsequently the other gentleman, Dr—— , saw the lady and concurred, and went so far as to say that delay, even till the next day was most dangerous for fear of constitutional infection.

My kind professional brethren impatiently scouted my views as mere senseless, not to say wicked, talk.

On examining the right breast and comparing it with the left, one was struck with the diminution in the size of right one. The nipple was deeply retracted, and from the little funnel-shaped opening in the nipple-region there oozed an ill-smelling fluid. The breast itself was puckered, and one raised ridge on it's outer aspect was inflammed, swelled, and bluish at one part,—an unmistakable picture of cancer. I therefore agreed as to the diagnosis.

We had a very long conversation about it, and it was a terrible position for me to take up in face

of almost all the experiences of the world in face
of the eminent authorities arrayed against me in
the teeth of the sneering, jeering opposition of
connexions, belongings; and their medical and
surgical friends.

Nor was it easy for the responsible friends or
the patient her self to decide finally either for my
treatment by the medicines or for the operation.

To see the unfortunate lady looking at her
sisters, then at me, then at her poor breast, and
then reading her doctor's letters urging the im-
perativeness of immediate operative interference,
and then bursting into a flood of tears, and saying
she did not know what to do, is a scene similar
to others I have often seen; but it remains ever
with me all the same. I concluded the delibera-
tions by saying "Mrs.—, the breast is *yours*; mark
that; not your sisters', not your doctors', not mine,
but yours; and if I were you I would *keep it*. I
promise you nothing, but I tell you that in my
experience, and speaking humanly, medicines can
cure you, though the course of the cure will be
slow; for that I find is almost invariably the case
in treatment of tumours, whether malignant or
benign, the mending by the help of medicines is
slow."

"Well," said she, "I refuse the operation, and

will do as you tell me."

The breast being painful (the weight of a heavy dog by it's paws), I ordered Bellis per. I, ten drops in water every four hours. This was April 2, 1887. Nothing locally at all, now, or hereafter.

April 1. Vast improvement.

Rx Arnica montana 1x. five drops three times a day.

April 21. Better on the whole.

Rx Repeat the Arnica.

April 28. Wakes with a nasty taste in the mouth.

Rx Repeat and also give *Chelidonium majus* 1x.

May 5. Not quite so well, and the skin of diseased breast is red; more painful; has just menstruated.

Rx Bellis per q. Five drops in water three times a day.

May 12. Better a good deal; the covering skin is less red, and the nipple is not quite so much retracted.

May 18. Mending beautifully; breast is softer; nipple less drawn in; a portion of the cutaneous covering is still red.

Rx Repeat.

May 26. Mending.

Rx Repeat.

June 2. The mammilla is less retracted, and the breast begins to be slightly movable. Heretofore it was so retracted and held down by bridles of tissue behind it that it could not be moved as a whole at all. Is menstruating.

Rx Repeat four times a day.

June 9. Still improving; nipple less retracted.

Rx Repeat.

June 16. The breast is getting bigger (i.e. returning towards it's previous natural size) and less immovable.

Rx Repeat five times a day.

June 23. The breast is much less drawn in; the top of the nipple is now sunk only about half an inch from the level; all the discoloration has gone from the mammary surface; and patient is getting stouter.

Rx Repeat.

July 2. Much running from the nose; runs

like water ever since she took the Bellis (Pathogenetic?). There is a little more tenderness of the breast; to-day the last day of the menses.

Rx   Repeat.

July 9. Some redness around the Areola mammillac.

Rx Repeat.

July 14. The coryza is very bad, for which patient comes; bad cough; much green expectoration tinged with blood. The cold is liked others she has had.

Rx Repeat.

July 28. The breast not quite so well (Is menstruating).

Rx Repeat gtt.x.

August 6. I learn to-day from the patient, for the first time that this right nipple has peeled at times for years with offensive discharge. In this state it is now.

Rx Repeat.

August 16. No change in the nipple, which is still peeling.

Rx Repeat.

August 25. The breast is slowly returning to the normal as to appearance, but there is still much discharge form the nipple.

Rx Repeat.

September 8. There is a little redness of the areola.

Rx Repeat Sul 30., three drams gtt. v. ter die.

September 27. Much improved, but the redness is there still.

To take Belladonna 30 with the Sul. and thereafter return to the Bellis as before.

October 11. Mending; the breast is slowly resuming it's former proportion, though it is still hard.

Rx Repeat Bellis θ.

November 12. Not so well.

Rx Hydrastis can. θ.

Now. 19. Slight improvement, there being less redness in the areola.

Rx Repeat.

Nov. 29. The Hydrastis seems to be causing diarrhoea.

Rx Arnica montana 3x.

December 8. Has a cold.

To alternate *Aconite* 3x with the *Arnica*.

Dec. 29. Breast continues hard, but there is less areolar redness.

Rx Chelidonium θ and Aconite 3x.

But I need not go on with these wearisome details; some more remedies were needed, patient got better and better, and returned early in 1888 to Germany, and I have not since seen her; but in a letter to me, under date of May 8, 1888, patient says "the hard lump is slowly decreasing." Perhaps before this goes to press I may be able to give the end of treatment, but this will not much matter, as patient was practically well before she left for the Continent.

I may add that the two English doctors who were so sure that it was cancer, and who insisted upon immediate operation, and whose letter I myself read when asked by me through the patient (just before she left for the Continent) whether they would allow me to have their original letters containing their diagnosis, prognosis, and recommendation of operation; well—they refused! And now they deny that they ever said positively that it was cancer; they only recommended the operation in case it should be cancer.

The frankness and honesty of one's allopathic colleagues are wonderful articles. However, they have, as usual, had to munch the leek. They great pity is that so much energy should be used up by us medical reformers merely to keep on our feet. We boast a good deal of our advanced state of culture and civilisation, but will some one explain to me how it is that many of even the most wonderfully cultured and most highly educated people of the day seem absolutely incapable of differentiating between self-denying, not to say heroic, medical reformers and persons who sell nostrums. In practical medicine this is crux indeed. But the world was ever thus.

TUMOUR OF BREAST

At the end of the month of November of the year 1886, a married lady of 40 odd years of age came to consult me in respect of a hard tumour of the size of hen's egg in the lower third of her left breast, painful at times, and due originally, it was stated, to a hurt. I find no note to the date of the hurt. Patient was the mother of large family, and she had also flooded and miscarried, and her menses had always been very profuse and long lasting, so that for year she had been barely ever able to completely recover from one period before she was overtaken by another, and hence she had acquired a weak heart from the chronic anaemia. She had suffered also for many years badly from leucorrhoea, and letterly her feet swelled. She was stated to have had scarlatina, measles, and mumps, each twice, and besides having had smallpox, she had been four times vaccinated, the last three times unsuccessfully. There were many little wartinesses here and there on the contineous surface, such as I have become accustomed to regard as pointing to cancer.

Rx Thuja occidentalis 30.

December 18. Very great improvement was reported, and patient was well of the tumour and of herself by the spring of 1887.

Beside the Thuja occid. Given repeatedly and over a number of weeks, Magnesia sul 3x was given the some little time. Over a year later the patient was reported to me as being well.

Here the medicinal and curative action was not only very remarkable but also very remarkably prompt, which attribute to the fact that the swelling was merely a dyscratic organismic reaction to the trauma of such recent date that the swelling was not yet neoplastic. When the casual dyscrasia was extinguished predisposing cause of the swelling was gone too, and hence the swelled tissue constituting the tumour had shrink shrivel. I thought it would have taken much longer to cure the tumour than it actually did, because it seemed to me probable that neoplasia had set into a greater extent than was evidently the case.

TUMOUR OF LEFT BREAST

At the beginning of 1888 I was consulted in regard to a tumour of the left breast of a healthy young lady of about 20 years of age, and which had not been noticed very long. It was in it's upper and outer aspect, but deep in the body of the breast. Of course, the young lady's mother and friends were greatly alarmed, and an operation was thought to be the only thing to do. It stands described in my account of case of the size of large orange, but I do not think it was quite so large. In four months the tumour had quite disappeared, the remedies having been, Thuja occidentalis 30, Bellis perennis θ, Ceanothus Americanus 1, and *Condurango* 1x, and the last named being apparently the remedial force, and which was given because of the browny look of patient's skin.

The rapid cure of this tumour was evidently

due to the fact that it was from reflected ovarian irritation, and not a neoplasm. Nevertheless it was only "an operation" that the faculty and family discuseed together indeed, the ready way in which the operating representative carpenters, commonly called surgeons, recommend the removal of ladies breasts in whole or in part is truly staggering.

TUMOUR OF RIGHT BREAST
IN A MAN

lthough tumours of the breast are much more common in women than in men still they do also occur in the breasts of males, more particularly in later life. Such a one is the following:-

On April 23, 1881, there came to me a rather tall, spare, cachectic-looking gentleman, a London professional man, of about 70 years of age telling me that ever since the previous February he had been greatly worried, and this was followed by a sensitiveness in his left nipple, which soon passed off and went to right nipple, wherein it still was. On examining the part I found it the seat of a hard tumid mass of the size of pigeon's egg. Patient first noticed it was swelled a month previously. It is not actually painful, but there is a sensation of fullness and uneasiness, and he cannot lie on it, hence it arrests his attention.

Rx Psor. 30. mvj.; s.1. q.s., ft. pulv., tales xij., j. nocte.

May 7. There is still a sensation of fullness in it; patient thinks it is softer, in which opinion I share. It is a little smaller. Since taking the powders he has had some bilious attacks.

Rx Repeat.

May 21. It is much smaller; there is much less sensitiveness, and patient can now sleep lying on his right side, which was previously not possible.

Rx Repeat.

May 28. The sensitiveness is now confined to the nipple alone, still he can sleep lying on it. He is constipated, and his tongue thickly furred.

Rx Hydrastis canadensis 3x, four drams.

S. gtt. v., nocte maneque.

June 14. The sensitiveness; tumour still continues, but it has very much distressed.

Rx Repeat.

July 2. Less sensitiveness; tumour still decreasing in size; on the sternum, on a level with the nipple, there is a scably eruption of the size of a three penny piece, having a red ground, the rest being yellowish. He is still constipated.

Rx Tc. *Hydrastis canad.* 3x four drams., s.gtt. v., n.m.

July 23. He has scabs on the scalp; a yellow scab at the middle of the sternum; also on his hands. The nipple is no longer sensitive at all.

Rx Tc. *Thuja occid.* 30, in infrequent doses.

August 13. The tumour has disappeared, with the exception of one of the size of a hazel-nut. There is still some scaly eruption on the sternum.

Rx Psor. 30 (two to a month).

Sep. 16. No. trace of the tumour to be found. There is still a patch of reddish scaly eruption on the skin of the chest.

Rx Tc. Chelidon maj. 3x, gtt. iij., nocte.

Oct. 13. No trace of tumour; still a circular patch at midsternum. Bowels a little relaxed.

Rx Trit. 6, Nat. sul.

Oct. 27. Well; and has a healthy complexion, whereas it was at the beginning of treatment, quite earthy.

Six years have elapsed since then, during all

which time the patient has remained well of the tumour, i.e., it has never returned. Two or three times or more in every year the gentleman is in the habit of coming to see me, "to be kept in repair." Before I began the treatment I was importuned by his friends as to whether I was quite sure it was safe to forego an operation, "which, you know, sir J——says is the only chance!"

What did the friend say after the tumour was cured by remedies? Were they grateful? Perhaps; they have so scrupulously avoided the subject ever since that I have no means of knowing.

Nevertheless the tumour remains cured, and that is the main point.

If any care to know my opinion of the pathology of this tumour, I wish to say I think it was scirrhus. That it was a very hard lump is quite sure.

Speaking biopathologically, more meo, the basis of the thing was PSORA-VACCINOSIS.

THE CAUSES OF TUMOURS OF THE FEMALE BREAST

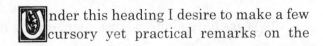

nder this heading I desire to make a few cursory yet practical remarks on the causation of mammary tumours in women. To begin with, the tumours in the female breast are very rarely primary to the breasts, but are most commonly produced in the breasts much in the same way that organ enabled to perform it's natural function of suckling the human off spring, i.e., the part is rendered physiologically active from the utero-ovarian sphere. Whether this views of the origin of mammary tumours has ever been promulgated before I do not know, in any case I have it from my own observations in practical life. Usually there is some disease or irritation in the lower part of the body, either arising primarily there or else expressed there holopathically. I will not enter into the details of these causes here, as the subject is too large for my present purpose, which will be sufficiently served if I say that wearing pessaries, taking intra-vaginal injections for the purposes of cleanliness or otherwise, or for the cure of mechanical hurts and injuries to the parts, the cautery, genesaic frauds and surrogates, all these may severally result in the formation to tumours in the ovaries, uterus, or breasts. The point I here insist upon is that mammary tumours do not usually arise from a cause existing primarily in the breasts themselves, but the cause is usually in some other more or less remote part of the organism, most frequently in the ovaries. Or the cause is organismic, and the tumour is the mammary expression of the constitutional condition of the individual.

And even where ;the tumour arises directly from a knock or below; or from pressure from the stays, there is usually something the constitutional crisis that favours neoplasms; and it is this something which constitutes the danger to the future integrity of the individual. If I am correct in what I here maintain with regard to the place of real primary origin and causation of tumour in the female breasts, then it must follow that operation can never be any cure since it is only the product that is operatively got rid of, and not the disease radically. In proof of this, see the number of cases which I relate even in this small volume, in which the disease returned in the other breast after it had been cut out of one. The number of the times in which I myself have seen this recurrence of tumours, after they had been got rid of by operation, is so great that I could adduce an absolutely overwhelming chain of evidence to prove this my contention, but I forbear; the fact is patent, and within the experience of all medical men, and, indeed, of almost all ladies of experience who take cognizance of what goes on in their own social circles.

I conclude, therefore, that both theory and

experience condemn the use of the knife, which is no cure for tumours. Is an operation, then, absolutely and always useless and damnable? No quite that, though it is not often needful if the case is taken early, when the tumour is young, as medicines can cure it vitally; BUT when it has become large—very large, broken, granulating, and auto-infective, then an operation is called for, but medicinal means should be at once used to prevent recurrence. In the earlier stages operation is damnable and dangerous.

I have ALREADY said that by tumours I understand all lumps and swellings whatever, the same being more or less growths on or in the human body, inclusive of such as are called cancer.

Woman's nature is essentially plastic, formative; wherefore woman is the mother of every man of us.

When woman's formative power becomes perverted by trauma, vice, or disease, it is apt to localize itself by creating a lump in the breasts or else where. Of course men get tumours also, but that is the reason of their being the sons of women, and possessing some of their formative power thus perverted and locally expressed.

Ten years or more ago Dr. pope, of Tunbridge

Wells, cured a lady of tumour with remedies chosen according to the homoeopathic law, and a friend of the cured one, having a tumour in her breast, sent for me to know if I could do for her what Dr. Pope had done for her friend. I found a tumour of breast about the size of an orange, hardish and irritable, and particularly trouble some at the period. The lady was young, for several years married, childless, and suffering from severe chronic leucorrhoea, which she was keeping in check by means of vaginal injections. The lady was very enthusiastic about the injections; they made her so comfortable, and they commended themselves to her judgement as a praiseworthy ablutionary measure.

Now, in the first place, I hold very strongly that mucous surfaces under natural conditions are not intended by nature to be washed, inasmuch as they are self-cleansing, and, in the next place, I maintain that diseases of the mucous membranes are for the most part constitutional, and should not be treated by local application.

I reason in this way: the mucous membrane is to the inside of the body just what the skin is to it's outside, and should be thus regarded physiologically and therapeutically.

Discharges from mucous surfaces are essentially much the same as eruptions on the cutaneous surface, and in the very deed are not infrequently identical.

And then Nature makes use of mucous surfaces from which to discharge peccant matter, of which she wishes to rid the economy. In ladies, the mucous lining of the vagina and of the womb are most convenient for this purpose, and hence the common occurrence of whites, which is it's expression.

Given a case of leucorrhoea, other than a temporary one, from a genuine cold or chill (when it's value is the same as a catarrh from the nose under like circumstances), and we have to deal with an affection of the organism, which it is dangerous to stop by local applications.

It is barely possibly to conceive of a case of chronic whites being local in nature and origin; it is a local expression of a constitutional cause in most cases.

With these views of the nature of whites, I explained to my patient that the tumour in her breast was caused, in my opinion, by the injections she was in the habit of using by way of cleanliness, and for the purpose of getting rid of the leucorrhoeal discharge. But as an eminent lady's doctor had recommended these said injec-

tions, maintaining that this leucorrhoea was a
merely local affair, the lady would not accept my
view of her case. Moreover, the local medical man,
of good standing in the profession, considered the
lump in the breast also a merely local affair of the
breast it self, and so the lady would also not accept
my view of the nature of this either.

Eminent medical authorities had declared to
her and to her husband that the leucorrhoea and
the lump in the breast had nothing to do with one
another, the discharge being merely an affair of
the vagina or womb, and the tumour being merely
an affair of the breast itself. Both husband and
wife ridiculed my view of the case, viz., that the
tumour was caused by the injections, and therefore I decided the case. Eight years later, a rela-
tion of their told me that this lady was still in very
ill-health, and that no one could do her any real
good.

Before leaving the question of the reciprocal
relations of the vaginal lining and the breasts, I
would like to refer to a very recent experience of
my own on the subject, as it tells the whole tale,
and that eloquently.

A married lady of 30, or thereabouts, and who
had formerly been under my care for phlegmasia
alba dolens, and hypertrophy of the spleen; came

quite recently to consult me in regard to a tume-
faction in her right breast. Having seen her about
her health only a very few months before, I was
really quite taken aback at her statement, and I
said, What have you been doing? "Oh, I went to
the seaside, and I there consulted the homoeopathic
doctor. Dr——, and he said my womb was retro-
verted, and he recommended me to wear a support, and after hunting me a good deal, and trying
five different sorts, one of which he called Hodge's
I was obliged to leave off trying as I could not bear
them. But before he put in the supports he found
that I had some ulcers of the womb, for which I
had to see him five times for something to be
applied to them. My breast began to trouble me
shortly after I returned home after undergoing
this treatment." I forbear to characterize either
the man or his treatment, but leave the facts to
speak for themselves. Of course, the patient was
duly recommended to his own special surgical
friend in town for the tumour of the breast, and
when I interposed and explained matters, the poor
lady cried and laughed in turns at being assured
that she would soon be quite well of the mammary
swelling without any operation.

By the way, we often find our operating
chirurgical carpenters tell in a very unctuous
manner of the beautifully ready way in which the

operated ones recover after the removal of a tumour, and they evidently seem to think that the quick healing of the wounds augnrs well for the furture of the case. But, as usual, their mental grip and positive knowledge are equal.

Dr. Moore, in his Manual of the Diseases of India, notes the curious fact that wounds heal remarkably quickly in the leper. This is interesting when coupled with the observation of Dr. Charles Creighton, that "amputations of the cancerous breasts have a peculiar tendency to heal by primary adhesion, as if the formative power in the several tissues were strong enough to dispense with the roundabout process of inflammatory reaction, suppuration, and reparative granulation."

Such, therefore, may be true value of the "healing skin". In fine, we may bear in mind in regard to the causation of tumours of the breast, when I think Kingsley somewhere thus expresses : "Outraged Nature is never tried of killing till she has taught man the terrible lesson he is slow to learn—that Nature is only conquered by obeying her.

"Nature is as fierce when she is offended as she is bounteous and kind when she is obeyed."

Now, just a word or two anent dietetic causes of tumours, and then I have done. In my experience they are—1. Much meat, notably pig meat; 2. Pepper and salt; 3. Milk; and in regard to this last named, no doubt many will be much amazed at my condemning the use of milk in tumours (particularly in those of the breast), but I do so most emphatically, and that from my own personal experience. Practical men would do well to remember this.

THE TREATMENT OF TUMOURS
BY MEDICINES

1. Having related enough cases of medicinal cures of mammary tumours to show that these tumours can be really got rid of with internal treatment, even when of a recurrent and cancerous nature, and having, moreover, made a few cursory remarks on their aetiology, it only remains for me to tell any younger or less experienced brother practitioners how to set about curding tumours with medicines. I have arrived at my present positive position slowly, gropingly, patiently, and quite independently; and I do not think I could do better than give very shortly my mode of procedure in principle. Where I asked to put down shortly my mode of setting about curing a case of tumour when it comes before me for medicinal treatment, I would say: First of all, I

begin by remembering Hahnemann's method of case-taking, and follow it partially; I say partially, because *time* is an element of importance nowadays.

2. Then I go over in my mind the various medical doctrines, such as those of psora, syphilis, sycosis vaccinosis, Grauvoglian constitutions and traumatism, not forgetting al the illnesses and diseases of the patient and any possible bearings of taints and dispositions, hereditary or acquired.

3. I take, then, a purely organopathic survey of the organ or part, and then weigh and balance the various facts which physiology, pharmacology, and pathology tell us about it.

When all this is done, I have usually at least one good reason for giving one good remedy which is then ordered, and which commonly teaches me the next step, either because it helps, or behaves indifferently, or otherwise.

Most commonly I find tumours are pathologically *hybrid* in their nature, and they will not yield to treatment of a simple nature, e.g., a person of the herpetic diathesis, who suffered much from gastric fever, was then vaccinated, then had much grief and sorrow, and finally had suffered from unrequired affection; and last of all, got a blow on her breast, followed by their formation to tumour, such a person in her very history tells the thoroughly competent therapeutist how to proceed without any symptomatology at all.

It has been urged against the homoeopahtic treatment of tumours that as the remedies used have (as a rule) never caused tumours or anything like them, and, moreover, are in all probability quite incapable of doing so, it must follow that there can be no real homoeo-therapeutics of tumours. This volume is a first part of my practical answer to this objection. It is brought out by itself for the reason already stated in my preface. I hope in a later publication to set forth in a clearer light my reasons for giving the remedies which I have found of greatest use in the treatment of tumours, some of which I have herein already referred to.

What I aim at in this volume is to prove that tumours can be truly and genuinely cured by medicines given by the mouth; and if I have proved that, then I have attained my object.

NEVERTHELESS, IN ORDER TO AID any younger practitioners in attempting the internal treatment of tumours, i.e., by remedies, I will just add a list of a few of the most useful medicines for this purpose, giving them alphabetically, with a practicalnote or two for the uninitiated. For further information, see Hughes's Pharmacody-namics* last edition, and back numbers of the *British Journal of Homoeopathy, of the Monthly Homoeopathic Review, and of the Homoeopathic World.*

REMEDIES USEFUL IN
TUMOURS OF THE BREAST

ad I the requisite leisure I could obtain from the medical literature of the world a mass of remedies that have been found useful in the cure of tumours in the various parts of the body : but there is this peculiarity about most of the cases of tumour published as cured by medici-nal means, that they are for the most part quasi-accidental, or, at any rate, extremely isolated; and one can read them ever so often, and any number of them, and still, when a case of tumour comes up for treatment, one finds that they have not given any particular clue to guide one.

I have already stated the way in which I set about curing tumours of the breast; and as I have mentioned under each case most of the; remedies used, I need not refer to those medicines here, but shortly to the following :- *Acidum aceticum* has a certain reputation for cancerous and benign tumours. Dr. J.C. Peters maintains that it will dissolve the "cancer cell." I have used it with advantage in cancer, but principally as an external irritant, notably in hepatic and pyloric indurations.

Aconitum napellus—The use of Aconite in tumours of the breast is by no means to be despised, as it commands congestion to some extent, which is a great help. Of course it has no direct or specific action.

Apis mel.—Of this remedy Dr. Gilchrist* (a very high authority) says :

"Apis mel.—I have frequently benefited, if not cured, various malignant and semi-malignant growths with the following symptoms :

Small ulcers with a gray slough, deep, and running into one another; pain, burning itching or stinging; sharp stinging pain in the ulcer or tumour; pus is of a light yellow colour, and scanty; erysipelatous inflammation of the surrounding skin; dark purple colour of old scars; thirst is either absent or increased for small quantities.

Worse in the morning; also from warmth ?

"*Better* from cold water and pressure. Left side.

"Has been used in many varieties of tumour, perhaps with a special adaptability to cystic formations. I have used it in cases of cancerous ulceration with good results a number of times you will find a case of ovarian tumour reported cured by this agent in the *North American jour. of Hom.*, vol. xxi., p 553, by Dr. Piersons; also one by Dr. P.H. Hale, in Raue's An. Rec.,1872, p. 173. In the latter case the 1st dilution was used, in the other the high. Dr. Garnsey, of Batavia, Ill., reports a case cured, in which he used *Apis* and *Apocyn.* Can. in alternation (Am.Hom. Obs., vol. iv., p. 251). In Helmuth's *Surgery,* p. 1181, a case is reported cured with the same remedy in alternation with Arsenic, reported by Dr. Craig. These two last cases are not as valuable as they might be, on account of the alternation of the remedies."

Apocynum cannabinum—It is a solvent unquestionably. I have thus cured a case of adenoma with it, used in the form of an ointment. It's action seems, in such cases, to be powerfully solvent.

Arnica montana—The great sphere of Arinca is trauma and haematoma. Dr. Lee cured a case of "movable" tumour of the orbit with it.

Argentum nitricum—It is sometimes useful in cutaneous cysts, and notably in the hydraemic.

Arsenicum—It is a classic remedy for bleeding cancer and many cases cured or ameliorated by it have been published. It has an equally great reputation for the cure of lupus.

Arsenicum iodatum—It has cured cancer of the breast, and also of the womb.

Aurum metallicum—It is useful in mammary indurations, particularly after mercury has been used.

Aurum muriaticum natronatum, taken by itself, is probably the best remedy for uterine tumours that we have.

Barium—It has a reputation for lipomata; the carbonate is used, and also the iodide and the muriate.

Belladonna—It is used by myself merely for it's congestive effects, and of course, in refracted dose it helps and relieves.

Bellis perennis—A very grand remedy, but, being only a common weed, is unknown or condemned and despised. It was ever thus. I have already illustrated its use in tumours of the breast.

Bryonia alba—It cured a case of fibroid tumour in the hands of Dr. C. Wesselhoeft. In my judgment, it is an important tumour medicine by reason of its demonstrated effects in arthritic states, and in circum-oophoritic peritonitis; and where the peritonium is probalby involved in the ovarian tumours, it will greatly relieve. The following note on line is from Gilchrist :

Calcarea carb.—Tumours occurring in the characteristic calcarea individual. Tendency to boils; to take cold easily; deficient animal heat; cold feet; perspiration of the feet and head particularly; pus is copious, putrid, yellowish,or white like milk; similar to Baryt. Carb., excepting that the subject are younger. Staph (Archives, vol. iii) reports a case of encephaloma of the eye, which; was cured after commencing the process with Calc. There is much doubt existing as to the correctness of the diagnosis Dr. Sumner (N.Y. Stater Hom. Mad. Soc. Trarns., vol. ix.) reports a case of ovarian tumour cured by this remedy. Prof. Beebe (World's Convension, 1876) reports a case from Helmuth of sebaceous cyst cured; Dr. Alvarez (Med. Invest, vol. iv., p 89) a case of lipoma; Prof. Beebe (loc.cit.) a case of fibrous tumour, in alternation with Coni, however, taken from Helmuth. I can report one case of uterine fibroid cured. A number of polypiexisted; the large ones were expelled, and the smaller disappeared by absorption. Nasal and uterine polypi have been cured so frequently that no citation of cases is necessary.

Calcarea phos.—The indications are similar to those under the carbonate. Perhaps there is a greater tendency to deficient ossification in the case of this remedy. I have thought that the Carbonica is of special value in cases of pedunculated fibroids; the Phosphate when sessile.

Condurango—The indications for this powerful drug have been already given.

Colocynthis—Gilchrist and Caroll Dunham have each recorded a case of ovarian cyst cured by this remedy. Sharp abdominal pains lead to its choice.

Conium maculatum—I have cured one case of tumour with this old favourite of Stoerk's, and it also has done me very good service in cancer of the tongue.

Ferrum—In the cachexia I have found Ferrum aceticum in small material dose of great benefit; in fact, I have often interrupted the more constitutional treatment for a little intercurrent course of iron, and with much advantage. Where there is plethora, of course a higher dilution must be used. I like Schussler's phosphate of iron. And the picrate, by reason of it's cephalic, hepatic, haemic, and local actions, is a grand remedy.

Galium ap.—Drs Bailey and Clifton have had brilliant results with this remedy in cancer of the tongue, particularly the latter, who has probably cured as many tumours by medicine as any living man.

Galium was used in combination with glycerine, the indication was evidently "Old Herball."

Graphites has a well merited reputation for wens and herpes and tumours in the herpetic.

Hydrastis canadensis—The late Dr. Bayes, had quite a reputation for tumours, and he set great store by it's use.

Poor Bayes, *in Brit. Jour. of Hom.* Once published the following list of cases treated with *Hydrastis canadensis*:-

Case	Age	Sex	Disease	Location	Result
1.	41	Female	Scirrhus.	Breast.	Cured.
2.	46	do	Cancer.	Right breast.	Much improved.
3.	77	do	do	do	Arrested.
4.	25	do	Scirrhus.	Cervical.	Much improved.
5.	45	do	do	Breast.	Pain relieved.
6.	50	do	Ulcerated cancer.	Left breast.	Greatly improved.
7.	37	do	Cancer.	do	Cured.
8.	48	do	do	Right breast.	Pain relieved.
9.	38	do	Tumours (cancerous).	Both breasts.	Much improved.
10.	48	do	Scirrhus.	Os uteri.	No. effect.
11.	56	do	Cancer— ulcerated	Os uteri, vagina, & rectun	do
12.	42	do	Scirrhus.	Uterus. do	
13.	60	do	Fungus haematodes.	Right thigh.	do
14.	22	do	Cancer.	Left breast.	Cured.
15.	50	do	Ulcerated cancer	do	Relieved.
16.	50	Male	do	Lip.	Arrested and improved.
17.	40	Female	Carcinoma	Left breast	Relieved.
18.	58	do	Scirrhus.	do	Arrested.
19.	40	do	Ulcerated cancer.	Os and cervix uteri.	Slight & temporary relief.
20.	60	do	do	do	No relief.
21	37	do	do	do	Arrested.

I, too, have used it a good deal and fully endorse Dr. Bayes views. Dr.Blake cured a case of epithelioma and also one of scirrhus with *Hydrastis.*

Iodine—It is not a favourite of mine indeed, I hardly know how to use it, as a nearly as one I see with a tumours has already had it in some form or other. However, I have used it in tumours of the pancreas with striking effect. (See Rademacher on this remedy in regard to this organ.)

Kali chloratum—It is a good remedy for mammary tumour that is little more than a mastitis.

Lappa major—I once knew a "Lady Bountiful" who used to cure poor people of swellings with a tea made of the roots of this plant. Her indication was—the blood.

Kali brom. Cured a case of ovarian tumour in the hands of the late Dr. Black.

Kali iod. Has been used with advantage in cases of supposed epithelioma. So has kreosotum.

Lapis alb.—The late Dr. von Grauvogl introduced this Urkalkgneiss for occult cancer, glandular tumours and bronchocele. He was led to use it by having observed the tumourifacient effect of the water containing it. Von Grauvogl sent me a portion to try some years before his death, with a very kind letter which I have preserved and still cherish.

Phosphorus—Has helped me in mammary tumours when given for menorrhagia, but I have generally used in the bleeding stage in alternation with Carb-animalis.

Phytolacca dec.—Is of undoubted value in mammary tumours, but requires to be given in material doses. In refracted dose I have found benefit from it in mammary atrophy; in one case, the increase in the size of the breasts was notable.

Platina and Pulsatilla are remedies to be remembered in mammary tumours, and also *Silicea, Acidum Fluoricum, Mercurius,* and many others.

I have myself obtained the greatest help from *theories* of drug action, diatheses,and specificity of seat as well as of action; and medicines that are known as mere organ-remedies will often cure it's organ of the disease that caused the tumour, and then the tumour atrophies.

Dr. Gilchrist, a surgeon of the right sort, i.e., one who places medicines first, in his small but important treatise on tumours and to which I have already referred, makes the following re-marks :-

"Prof. Helmuth, in his paper on 'The Influence of Homoeopathy upon Surgery,' And Prof. Beebe, in one upon 'The Therapeutics of Benign Tumours,' presented to *World's Homoeopathic Convention* in 1876, held in Philadelphia, refers, at some length, to a large number of doses in addition to those I have presented. To the student I recommend a study of there papers.

"In all forms of tumour I have now referred to one hundred and thirty-two cases reported cured. *All* of these cannot be fraudulent, incorrect, or of doubtful diagnosis. Indeed, as tumours differ, in these classes, mainly in a plus or minus of cellular elements, it can make but little difference whether the exact form is correctly diagnosticated or not. The fact of it's being a tumour at all is the all-important question. Large as this list of cures is, it might readily be extended, but those who doubt would continue to do so if volumes were written."

THE POST-PROVING SPHERE OF DRUG ACTION IN RELATION TO THE THERAPEUTICS OF TUMOURS

One very great almost insurmountable, difficulty in the homoeotherapeutics of tumours, lies in the inadequacy of our homoeopathic provings, which are not carried far enough to produce hypertrophy of degraded tissue, and usually not even far enough to degrade the tissue. And indeed it may be questioned whether it would be justifiable to prove remedies on ourselves sufficiently long to set up such an organic process.

But, according to the Roman proverb, we may learn of the enemy. And article in the June (88) number of the Monthly Homoeopathic Review is here trenchantly interesting, and I therefore will not be withhold it:

ARSENIC AND CANCER

t a meeting of the Pathological Society in December last. Dr. Jonathan Hutchinson made a communication on arsenical cancer of which the following abstract appeared in the British Medical Journal on the ensuing Saturday :

"Arsenic Cancer—'Mr. Jonathan Hutchinson, F.R.S., desired to make the internal administration of Arsenic in large doses over long periods might produce a form of cancer which was of the epithelial variety, but presented certain peculiarities. He showed a drawing of the foot of a gentleman who had taken Arsenic for psoriasis for many years; a corn on the sole of the foot ulcerated, and at first had the appearance of perforating ulcer. Perfect immobility was not followed by any improvement. The palms of the hands also became affected, small corns developing. The growth in the foot was excised and the patient recovered. The patient was now under the care of Professor Chiene; the Microscopical examination was inconclusive. He also showed drawings of the hands of an American physician who had taken Arsenic for long periods in considerable doses. A rough condition of the palms and soles developed though the psoriasis was cured. These early growths in the observed, parenthetically, were corns, not warts, and the growths were never papillary. This patient then got on the front of the wrist of the left hand a growth in the subcutaneous tissue, the other hand also became affected; the growths perforated the skin and fungated; they had the appearance of a syphilitic lesion, but the patient had never had that disease. The growths were scraped away and also excised; microscopical examination was again at first inconclusive, but the opinion finally leaned to the view that the disease was cancer. The patient then came to Europe, and in deference to the opinion of several surgeons, antisyphilitic remedies were fairly tried, but gave no result. Both hands were amputated;

the patient died eighteen months later. Nodules of epithelial cancer were found in the axillary glands on the left side, in both lungs, in the suprarenal capsules, in a rib, and in other parts. He also showed drawings from another case of a lesion of the palms, exactly resembling the corns seen in the other cases. This patient had a cancerous growth in his neck, and took Arsenic in large doses, for months together; the skin became muddy and thick, and patches like psoriasis developed upon the elbows and other parts, but in the palms and soles the corny masses formed, but were not followed by cancer. About five years ago, Dr Clifford Allbhtt had given him the particulars of a case of a young lady who had taken Arsenic for pemphigus for many years, with occasional intermissions. An ulcer had developed on the crest of the ilium the glands enlarged, a tumour formed in the thigh, and the patient died at the age of 25, owing to the enlargement of these growths. Mr Hutchinson also mentioned a case which had been under the care of Mr. Waren Tay and himself. The patient was a clerk, aged 34, who had taken Arsenic for a long time for psoriasis. The palms of his hands and soles of his feet were speckled over with corns when he applied at the Skin Hospital; finally, epithelial cancer of the scortum appeared, and was excised; the patient was then lost sight of. He thought the facts he had brought forward warranted him in advancing the theory that the cancer in these cases was due to Arsenic, with hope that attention might thus be more generally directed in the point.

"In the discussion which followed, Dr. W.B.Hadden mentioned that he had seen several cases of erythematous eruptions in children with chorea taking Arsenic. Mr Eve said that he believed that epithelial cancer of the palms always presented peculiar apperarances, which agreed with those described by Mr. Hutchinson, and added that lymphosarcoma of the lungs occurred with considerable frequency in workers in cobalt mines, a fact which he thought lent support to Mr Hutchinson's theory. The President (Sir James Paget, Bart.,F.R.S.) said that he had seldom heard an argument, founded on clinical and pathological evidence, more definitely suggesting the conclusion advanced. In this connexion it must be remembered that chronic psoriasis was sometimes followed by cancer. In the face of the facts advanced by Mr Hutchinson, it could not, he felt, be doubted that Arsenic had a power, in persons predisposed to it, to determine the development of cancer. The first two cases he had seen himself, and he had been clearly of opinion that the disease was cancerous. Mr. Hutchinson, in reply, remarked that microscopical evidence in the early stages of cancer was often conflicting and misleading. For instance, in this American case many most competent pathologists, both in England and on the microscopical specimens, formed the opinion that the growths were not cancerous, yet the patient undoubtedly had cancer, and had died of it. He believed that herpes zoster was certainly produced by Arsenic; Arsenic eczema had already been described. A remarkable fact about Arsenic eruptions was that they were never symmetrical.

"The only lesson that the members present, when Mr. Hutchinson made this communication, would learn from it would be that they should be more cautious in prescribing *Arsenic* in the future, this, indeed, is admitted by *The Lancet* in it's enusing number. To those members of this profession who have learned by experience that Hahnemann's therapeutic rule-*similia similibus curantur*—is indeed the bridge that spans the gulf so long fixed between the pharmacologist labouring to elucidate the mysteries of the subtle actions of drugs upon the complicated and intricate human organism, and the therapeutist struggling to apply these results to the successful treatment of disease (*British Medical Journal,* August 9th, 1884), it had a far higher value, Perhaps we should rather say that it you have had such a value, were it not for the fact that the study of the symptoms of chronic arsenical poisoning had long since taught us the importance of *Arsenic* in the treatment of cancer. Long previous to Hahnemann's time, *Arsenic* was an empirical remedy in cancer. But the selection of this drug by the light of the rule of similars has enabled us to differentiate those case of cancer which are most surely benefited by it from those in which it is less efficacious. Thus, Dr Dudgeon, in his article on *Arsenic* in The *Hahnemann Materia Medica,* part I p. 24 (1852), writes :-'It merely, palliates true scirrhus and medullary tumours; it is, however, curative in cancroidal tumours, as Dr. Bennett calls them, or, according to Mr. Paget, "epithelial tumours" So, too, Dr. Hughes says *Paharmacodynamics,* p. 261 4th ed., 1880), 'in epithelial cancer—as of the lip, face, and tongue—Arsenic has unquestionably proved curative, and that not seldom. Lastly, Dr. Pope, in a lecture on *Arsenic (Monthly Homoeopathic Review,* vol. xxx., p. 414), writes : 'In some cases of cancer Arsenic is, by the peculiar character of it's influence on the quality of th blood, as well as by the symptoms of general constitutional adynamia it produces, and the local burning and ulceration it excites, well indicated and often useful......It is in epithelioma that *Arsenic* can be prescribed with greatest advantage.

"Our selection, then, of *Arsenic* as remedy in cancer has been mostly confined to the epithelial variety of the disease. We have in Mr. Hutchinson's contribution an illustration of it's producing a condition exceedingly similar to this form of the disease-so much so, that Mr. Eve remarked that 'epithelial cancer of the palms always presented the peculiar appearances which agreed with those described by Mr. Hutchinson;' while Sir James Paget stated that 'it could not be doubted that *Arsenic* had a power, in persons predisposed to it to determine the development of cancer.'

"Our contemporary, *The New York Medical Record,* in referring to Mr. Hutchingson's paper, and 'his belief that Arsenic may produce, or at least be an exciting cause of epithelial cancer,' and after stating that 'Sir James Paget held the same view,' adds, this will be joy ful news to our homoeopathic brethren.'

"We certainly are glad to find our opponents, more especially such as have in years gone by been known to us as particularly bitter opponents, confirm the truth and accuracy of your drug pathogenesis by observations of their own. Let us now suggest to them to test the value of our therapeutic application of your pathogenetic observations, by giving Arsenic as a remedy in cases of epithelial cancer."

Let these wise words conclude my little volume on Tumours of the Breast, and their Treatment and Cure by Medicines.

**A wide variety of Books on the following subjects
by Indian and Foreign Authors are
also available with us:**

- Acupressure and Reflexology
- Acupuncture
- Aroma Therapy
- Astrology and Palmistry
- Ayurveda and Herbal Medicine
- Bach Flower Remedies
- Biochemistry
- Crystal and Gem Therapy
- Dowsing - Pendulam
- Feng Shui
- Health Care
- Holistic Medicine
- Homoeopathy

- Hypnosis
- Iridology
- Juice and Food Therapy
- Magnetotherapy
- Medical Dictionary
- Nature Cure
- Pet Animals
- Pranic Healing
- Reiki and Spiritualism
- Tai Chi
- Tarot
- Urine Therapy
- Vaastu
- Yoga

A detailed catalogue of books is available